The Gift of Cancer

my greatest teacher

Patsy McLean

Copyright © 2014 The Gift of Cancer: my greatest teacher

Published by BurmanBooks Media Corp.
260 Queens Quay West
Suite 1102
Toronto, Ontario
Canada M5J 2N3

All rights reserved. No part of this publication may be reproduced, stored in a retrieval system, or transmitted in any form by any process—electronic, photocopying, recording, or otherwise—without the prior written consent of BurmanBooks Media Corp.

Cover design: Lara Vanderheide
Cover Photo: www.CallbackHeadshots.com
Interior design: Lara Vanderheide
Editing: Nicolette Hernandez

Distribution:
NewLeaf Distribution
401 Thorton Rd.
Lithia Springs, GA 30122-1557

ISBN: 978-1-927005-39-2

Printed and bound in The United States of America

DISCLAIMER:

This book details the author's personal experiences and practical learning. The content provided is for general information purposes and should not be construed as medical advice. Please always remember to contact your healthcare provider to discuss any changes you are considering.

CONTENTS

Introduction:	Cancer, a Gift?	8
Chapter 1:	Life before my "detour"	10
Chapter 2:	What is Melanoma?	19
Chapter 3:	Surgery, Recovery and Results	25
Chapter 4:	But I was so healthy. How could this happen to me?	36
Chapter 5:	Stress – A Silent Killer	50
Chapter 6:	Digestion and Elimination	68
Chapter 7:	Food Comparisons – Then and Now	73
Chapter 8:	Juice and Smoothie Ideas for Detox and Healing	105
Chapter 9:	Recipe Ideas for Optimal Health	125
Chapter 10:	Toxins and Chemicals Everywhere?	177
Chapter 11:	The Exercise and Disease Connection	199
Chapter 12:	Q & A with Dr. Selene Wilkinson, ND	209
Conclusion:	What's Next?	214

Acknowledgements

Writing this book has been quite the adventure. I never realized how much goes into the process of completing a book. I'm so thankful to have so many wonderful people who supported me through this truly rewarding experience.

I would like to offer special thanks to my sister, Sandra, for her never-ending love, support and strength during this journey. My sincere thanks to Dr. Selene Wilkinson, ND for her powerful words of encouragement that changed the course of my life and her incredible ability to somehow make everything okay when challenges arise. I would like to thank my wonderful family for all the love and support they always offer. Thanks to Sandy and Petra, for being with me on surgery day and the post-surgery PJ party. Thank you Garnet for sharing your incredible energy. Thank you Amie, Cathy, and Emily for taking time to proofread and provide feedback. Thank you Jill, for sharing your delicious recipes. Thanks to Carolyn, for being my sounding board and amazing personal editor. My gratitude to Lisa Marie, for saving the day with the final chart edits. I would like to thank my colleagues and friends, for their continued support and encouragement from start to finish. Thanks to Nicolette for her incredible editing and calm understanding of my frustrations. I would like to thank Sanjay for pulling it all together. I could not have done this without all of your support.

Patsy

FOREWARD BY DR. SELENE WILKINSON, ND

I am very happy to have worked with Patsy during this challenging time in her life. Patsy's determination to regain her health was very inspiring to many people. Her story encourages others to recognize how our daily choices affect the state of our health and wellness. Patsy's commitment to the cancer protocol was 100%. She made a complete change in her choices immediately and continues to live with awareness. This book has lots of valuable information and reference tools. I look forward to continuing to see Patsy inspire others for many years to come.

Introduction: Cancer, a Gift?

How could anyone call cancer a gift? It's such a horrible disease.

Yes, it is. But it truly was a major teacher for me.

After my diagnosis and five years of researching and learning, I realized that I had many "health teachers" in my life. I chose not to listen to them or wasn't ready to hear them out. Maybe if I did at the time, it could have prevented my final diagnosis.

My own body

In my late twenties I had my gallbladder removed. I was told this was simply hereditary, since several family members have had the same surgery. I went on with life the same way I always did, not realizing this was a crucial opportunity to look at the true health of my body. I now know having a gallbladder removed was not hereditary. It was due to poor nutrition, high stress, and too much alcohol consumption. Yes, I was very successful, "living the good life", owning a business, a house, and two cars all before the age of thirty. I didn't realize what "the good life" was doing to my body.

Ina

I had a wonderful client, Ina, who offered me many opportunities to grow. During our long conversations, she shared tips from her experiences with relationships, investing, cooking tips, and spirituality. We even debated politics and news events. She always had the best of intentions when she shared her opinions and tried to encourage different ways of thinking and living. She was a person I could be completely open with, and I never felt judged for how I lived my life.

At the time, Ina was in her fifties, and was very strong and healthy. Her lifestyle was completely different than mine; she ate a vegetarian diet with lots of dark, green, leafy veggies, practiced meditation, went for long walks daily, and later became a yoga teacher. I joined her for a few yoga/meditation classes and was always open to hear about a new healthy food she had discovered. Yet, I always reverted back to my typical life as a young adult in my mid-twenties – high protein (keeps you lean), eating food-on-the-go (no time for cooking), frequent high- intensity exercise (to look great), work long hours (be successful), and late nights indulging myself with numerous alcoholic beverages (having fun). I looked up to Ina in so many ways, but at the time I just didn't understand how valuable the information was that she was offering me.

Now, the tips that Ina shared with me are part of my daily routine. I eat healthy, take long walks, exercise and meditate. I regularly practice yoga and hope to become a yoga teacher over the next year!

There were several "teachers" in my life that recognized the signs of my deteriorating health, and tried to suggest changes, but I wasn't ready. It wasn't until the next teacher was so great, I didn't have a choice, but to change.

Cancer was the gift of learning for me.

I share my story with you in hopes of preventing the necessity of a similar teacher appearing in your life. I now understand the importance of self-care and the special people who appear in our lives to show us the way. Material things are just that, *things*. Our body truly is our temple. Without our health, does anything else matter?

Chapter 1

Life before my "detour"

2005, the start of an amazing growth period in my life.

I had a very successful accounting business for over 15 years and loved everything and everyone involved with it. Fitness had always been a regular part of my life, but it had changed over the years due to long work hours. Setting up a gym in my home guaranteed my early morning routine to stay fit, but I was missing the fun and human interaction that comes with team sports and working out with others.

As I approached a milestone birthday I wanted a new goal to renew my commitment to exercise and team events. I decided to do something really special just for me. For my 40th birthday, I took on the challenge to run a half marathon in Barbados with the Leukemia and Lymphoma Society of Canada (LLSC). I trained regularly, and raised $6,000 to help those fighting blood cancers. I had never really done any volunteer work before and I wanted to do something special for others. I wanted to give back and celebrate my good fortune and good health at the age of 40.

So, off I went to Barbados! Even though I was a regular runner, I was not prepared for the hot weather, and struggled with a cramp right up to the finish line. But I finished! It was definitely a memorable birthday.

The trip was the start of several changes. When I returned home, the Leukemia & Lymphoma Society of Canada (LLSC) told me that they were developing a new "mentor" program to help motivate new runners. This meant running every Saturday morning with the group, answering questions, helping with fundraising, travelling to some events with the participants, and generally motivating them every step of the way.

After mentoring for almost a year, I decided to pursue a personal training certification so I was more prepared to assist the LLSC runners and for my own general interest. Approximately three months after the successful completion of my written and practical exams, the instructor of the course contacted me about a coaching position available for HBC Run for Canada. I accepted the position. It would be three nights a week, coaching employees from three different HBC locations for three months in order for participants to safely and successfully complete a 10km run.

It was such a rewarding experience! There were runners who had never run before and some who had completed the run the year before, who wanted to improve their time. Everyone was successful and I ran to the finish line with almost every participant that day. One girl even improved her time by 10 minutes! I received so many e-mails from the participants, thanking me and sharing their feelings after the race. It was incredible. I knew at that moment, big career changes were on the horizon.

In March of 2006, I had an accounting contract up for renewal. I did not renew it. I took a risk and pursued my passion: a career in fitness. By June 2006 I had 2 job offers. I accepted a position with the best club in Toronto! *Yes, I'm a little bias*. After two interviews, The Adelaide Club offered me a job with the requirement that I complete a post-rehab certification as a Medical Exercise Specialist. The doctor from California who teaches this course just happened to be running his annual 5-day course in Toronto in just two weeks! Coincidence? I think not. I completed the course, started working at the club, and studying for the exam.

Since I had a business background, there were times when I was surrounded by books and paper sitting on my couch thinking to myself, "Why did I ever think I could do this?"

Anatomy, medical terms, injuries, and hip/knee replacements were all new territory for me compared to my previous studies. After months of studying, I passed the exam, and secured my position. Wow, it was tough.

Everything happens for a Reason, Season, or a Lifetime.

Unknown

Life was perfect. I was developing my client base at the club, while still maintaining some accounting clients. I was just a little reluctant to give up all the security of my financial world. After all, it was all I'd known for over 15 years.

2009 – More Changes ahead

In spring of 2009, I was settled and thrilled to be working in the health and fitness field....but I wanted it to be full-time. I started looking at options that would allow me to utilize my business and training skills and help me move into a management position within the industry. Although I had successfully received over five certifications by this time, I didn't have the Kinesiology credentials that most have, so I thought I would go a different route. I heard about a fitness director position on a cruise ship. Although I would sacrifice nine months away from family, friends, and the job I loved, I could gain the experience I thought I needed. Besides, I love to travel.

I applied for the job and set up an interview for Aug 2009. I was excited, curious, nervous, and hopeful. At the same time, I was organizing a boot camp destination retreat for Sept 2009 in Santa Monica, California. This kept my mind occupied and off the "what ifs" of getting the job. The destination retreat was going to be the first one I've lead, with 6 ladies and I wanted it to be awesome.

In July 2009, I noticed a little bump on the left cheek of my buttocks. I'm very aware of my body, so I knew that it was something that had not been there before. I kept an eye on it for two weeks, thinking it was probably from running and sweating, since it was summertime. When it didn't go away, I went to my Doctor to ensure it wasn't something to worry about. She confirmed that it was a mole, *but it did not look suspicious.* When I told her about the boot camp I was planning in California, she thought it would be best if we removed it after I got back to prevent any chance of infection from the incision. I felt much better and went on with planning my Santa Monica boot camp.

After a phone interview for the cruise ship position, I completed the official interview on September 1st and I felt it went really well. I would find out in early September if a new job was in my future.

Now I was off to California for a week of exercise and fun with a fabulous group of women. Santa Monica was the perfect place for a boot camp. We stayed right on the beach beside the pier with quick access to the 26-mile bike path. This allowed us to run, bike, and rollerblade along with the daily boot camp workouts. We also spent a day horseback riding through the Santa Monica mountains. It was absolutely beautiful!

Half way through the trip I received the job offer for the cruise ship position. I was thrilled to accept the position and ready to start preparing for this new adventure, but I have to admit I was also a little scared. There had already been a major career shift in the past few years that I was now feeling like I didn't know where I belonged. I never shared this with anyone since they were always excited and envious of my life. Yet, as fun as my life appeared, there was always a deeper connection missing. I didn't recognize this at the time as a potential for disease, but looking back I see the need for constant change as a longing for something more meaningful. I became really good at hiding my emotions after the end of a long-term relationship several years before. Although always very driven, I think my career was also a way of not dealing with those deeper feelings. When emotions get buried they eventually find another way of expressing the feelings...like disease.

Everything happened so fast after I returned home from the trip. The cruise company booked me on a flight in late October to London, England to start my official training. I was ready for the next phase of life.

On Sept 17, 2009 I had my previously scheduled doctor's appointment to remove the mole from my left buttocks. I told my doctor about my new job and she was very excited for me.

One week later I received a call from the Doctor's office that she needed to see me. I was very surprised and I knew it had to be that silly little, "non-suspicious" looking mole. I arrived at her office two hours later to find out that I had Malignant Melanoma, the deadliest form of skin cancer.

I'm a pretty calm, non-emotional, factual kind of person so my immediate reaction was "Okay, so what are the next steps?"

My doctor was clearly in shock that this had happened to me, as I had very few "identified" health issues (except the Gallbladder) during my life and was very fit. She had me scheduled in to see a specialist the following week to start the ball rolling with a plan.

My life came to a screeching halt. I called my sister Sandra, who is my rock, on my way home. I remember saying to her "I'm not sure how I feel about this", I guess I was in a bit of shock. She just listened (like she always does) and let me start to process. She never reacted in a negative way. She just simply let me talk.

Sandra is such a strong woman in so many ways, and has always been there for me. We've shared many of life's ups and downs together. I've cried on her shoulder, talked for hours, shared thoughts and feelings that no other person knows about me. We can laugh for hours. She's the strong silent type. Just the type of person you need in a situation like this.

After processing this information overnight and researching melanoma on the computer, I was beginning to get concerned, but was still unemotional, until I was at work the next morning and went out to get a coffee.

I ran into our company Naturopath, Dr. Selene Wilkinson, the most amazing naturopath in Toronto. She said, "Hi, how are you?"

I cracked right there and then. I started to cry and said, "Selene, I'm not well. I have cancer." Her immediate response was incredible, she said, "Patsy you are strong, there is so much we can do."

I will never forget those words because right there, in that moment, she gave me back my power. It had momentarily been taken away by the word, Cancer. It's a word that can shatter your life and Selene is the person that helped me look at it very differently. She brought this gift of learning to my attention. I saw her later that day and she gave me a cancer food protocol to follow. I have to admit, I had no idea what some of the healthy food items were. Burdock Root? Never heard of it before....

I recruited my friend Tanya (who loves to cook) to go shopping with me the next day to show me where to find all the ingredients for the special soup I needed to make. I followed that protocol for the next year without fail. If it was not on my sheet, it did not enter my mouth.

I never looked at cancer as a death sentence for me. With Selene's help, I stayed present and didn't get caught up with "what if." My strong focus and determination had always been an asset in my career and was a great strength in my quest to regain my health. My health became my new "career." This started me on a journey of self-awareness, learning about toxins in our food, and chemicals in our world.

I had been training one of the girls who participated in the California boot camp for her very first half-marathon and despite what was going on in my life, I was not going to let her down. So three days after diagnosis, I ran 21.5km with her and she did amazing! We celebrated her accomplishment with lunch joined by some of the other California Boot Camp girls. At the end of our lunch, I shared the news.

These ladies were a huge source of support during the coming months. Our friendship grew out of my boot camp classes two nights a week. They would all arrive at my condo to drop off their backpacks, pickup a skipping rope/resistance band and off we'd go to the park to workout.

Even when I decided not to continue, as I wanted to infuse my body with nutrients and do my own specific workouts, they still all met at my condo and did boot camp at the park together. They were so encouraging every time I saw them. I was still able to hear all the funny life stories that we would usually share while at the park. It was so amazing to see this group of ladies, who met because of my boot camps, develop such a strong friendship and love of exercise. This confirmed why I do what I do!

My first meeting with the specialist was a dose of reality. His first comment to me was "So, you use a tanning bed." This was not a question. It was a statement. I told him I had used a tanning bed, but not on a regular basis. However, the last time I had used one I had experienced a terrible burn on my butt. I had not used a bed in several years, and did not realize how strong they had become over that period of time. The burn was bad.

His response was, yes that would do it. Wow, one bad burn from a tanning bed and now my life was about to change forever.

While all this was going on, I was still working and the only people who knew were Sandra, Selene, a couple of close friends, the boot camp girls, some clients and my bosses Dean and Blair. They had all been very supportive and understanding of what changes the coming months might mean for me both work and personally. I didn't share the news with everyone as I wanted to go on with my life as normal as possible and not have people constantly asking me how I was or looking at me with concern. My thought was, "It is what it is and I will deal with each day as it comes."

Not having to talk about it regularly allowed me to not think about it during my busy days. I did my processing at night.

I wanted to be able to tell my family members in person, so I decided to wait until Thanksgiving. The word cancer can instill such fear in people and I wanted them to see I was doing great and would move past this.

When I arrived, everyone was there, my parents, siblings, nieces, and nephews who were all excited to hear about my plans to move and start my training for the cruise ship in London, England. Did I have everything organized with my condo? When was my flight? Did I know what ship I would be on? My response was, "I'm actually not going to London right now as I have a little medical issue to deal with."

I just refused to get caught up in negativity and self-pity. *Thanks to Selene's powerful words.* When asked what the medical issue was, I simply said "It's not a big deal, so don't get all worried, but I have a little bit of cancer."

All said with a smile on my face and *looking* the picture of health. Of course, there was shock and concern, but I think my delivery and positive attitude kept everyone from thinking the worst. It's not something any family member wants to hear, especially parents, and I was determined to help them process the news, just as Selene had helped me.

My first consultation with the surgeons at Princess Margaret Hospital was an interesting day. I had a doctor from Israel and a doctor from Asia meet with me. Princess Margaret attracts the best, so I felt I was in good hands. They checked everything out and both felt that I was a low risk for the possibility of metastasis (spreading to other areas). Having said that, they still needed to take a big chunk out of my left buttock (about the size of an apple). Hey, what woman wouldn't love a little butt reduction? I joked with the doctors and said "Can you take a chunk out of the right butt cheek too? I want to keep them even," and I laughed.

One of the doctors didn't find me amusing. He said, "Melanoma is a very serious disease."

I gave a little chuckle and said "Don't worry, I know that. I'm just trying to stay positive and not get pulled into the negativity."

Positivity and laughter was obviously my coping mechanism, but deep down I really did know the seriousness of this diagnosis. I had done a lot of research. I had always been a "strong woman", easily dismissing feelings that could be viewed as weak, so it was difficult for me to show my real feelings to others.

The doctors told me I had to have a procedure called Sentinel Lymph-node removal. On the morning of the surgery, they would inject the cancer site with radioactive material that would follow the body's fluid to the first lymph-node. They would remove it and test to see if the cancer had spread to any other lymph-nodes that would need to be removed. In my case, the Sentinel lymph-node was in the groin area. Little did I know that this would be one of the most painful procedures I would ever experience. Deep breathing would be required for each of the four injections around the cancer site. After the injection, I would be able to watch the screen on the machine as a blue light, identifying the radioactive fluid as it started to move to show where the fluid was travelling and the location of the Sentinel lymph-node. The attendant would mark that area on my skin so the surgeon would know where to cut. Technology is quite amazing.

Before I left their office they gave me instructions and the date of surgery, November 9, 2009. In a few weeks it would all be over. One thing I was acutely aware of each time I went to Princess Margaret was how many people pass through there each day to receive chemotherapy treatments. It really makes you realize how important your health is and how prevalent cancer is in our world.

Chapter 2

What is Melanoma?

Melanoma isn't taken as seriously as it should. Melanoma is the deadliest form of skin cancer. One of my clients told me that someone she knew had recently passed away from Melanoma at the age of 29. Yes, 29. Diagnosed in February and passed away in August. I've read several sad stories like this since I started my research. Melanoma is deadly if not caught early. I was very lucky and this is why I believe my cancer was a gift, so I can share as much information as possible with you to help reduce your potential risk.

Melanoma diagnosis will continue to grow each year. American Cancer Society statistics predict that there will be 76,100 new cases of Melanoma this year and 9,710 people will die of Melanoma, which is preventable by some lifestyle changes.

What is your lifetime risk of getting Melanoma?

1 in 50 – Caucasian

1 in 1000 – Black skin

1 in 200 – Hispanic

In addition to the above, your risk **increases** if you have:

Fair hair (blonde/red) and light eyes (blue/green)

Weakened immune system

Large amounts of moles from sunburns over the years

I was surprised to learn from the Canadian Skin Cancer Foundation that skin cancer is the *most common type of cancer* and the most preventable. Until I was diagnosed, I didn't really know much about skin cancer. 1 in 3 cancers diagnosed worldwide is skin cancer, 80-90% of them are caused by ultraviolet radiation from either the sun or indoor tanning. I believe it's also the most misunderstood and dismissed cancer, as skin is not thought of as being an organ. Skin is actually an organ and, in fact, is the largest organ of the body.

I remember thinking a great tan made me look so healthy, but the damage can be so much greater than we realize. There are over 80,000 cases of skin cancer diagnosed each year in Canada and more than 5,000 cases are Melanoma. Melanoma is the deadliest form where patients potentially die within months of diagnosis. Imagine given news that you have only months to live and that it could have been prevented with lifestyle changes?

The changes I will share with you are not severe, but they do require consistency and commitment. These lifestyle modifications can save your life. Change does not mean giving up the sun or vacations. I still love to travel and I travel as often as I can to warmer climate. I don't spend hours in the sun trying to get dark skin in 1 week though. I stay covered with clothes or natural sunscreen, but I still enjoy the outdoors as often as possible.

Canadians born in the 1990's are two to three times more likely to get skin cancer (1 in 6) than those born in the 1960's (1 in 20).

That's something to think about the next time you want a "healthy tan."

THERE ARE 3 TYPES OF SKIN CANCER

BASAL CELL CARCINOMA, 80% of all skin cancer

Occurs in the lowest layer of Epidermis. The basal layer contains approximately 95% basal cells. This type of skin cancer is most common in the head and neck area. It is usually slow growing over time and rarely becomes more of a concern.

SQUAMOUS CELL CARCINOMA, 16% of all skin cancer

Occurs in the middle layer of Epidermis. This skin cancer is more aggressive than Basal. It is usually found on the hands, head, neck, lips, or ears.

MELANOMA, 4% of all skin cancer

Melanocytes make up approximately 5% of the Basal layer. This type of skin cancer is the most concerning with a high risk of death within 5 years if not found early.

According to the International Agency for Research on Cancer, there is a higher risk of Subcutaneous Melanoma by 75% when using tanning beds before the age of 30.

If Melanoma spreads, it is typically to the Liver, lungs, bones or brain.

It still boggles my mind how tanning beds can still be in business. Melanoma can show up anywhere on the body. So, unless you're regularly checking your skin for changes, it can be growing without being exposed until it's in the later stages.

There are four different types of Melanoma and specific signs that identify each. Health Central describes them as follows:

Lentigo Maligna Melanoma

This type occurs most often in older people with skin that has been damaged by the sun, in areas such as the face or hands. It may resemble a light brown or black freckle with a central nodule.

Superficial Spreading Melanoma

This type extends across the skin horizontally before invading the body. One may notice an irregular patch of skin in shades of black, gray, red, tan, blue or white.

Acral-Lentiginous Melanoma

This type is the least common form of melanoma. It appears as a black discoloration on palms, fingers, soles and toes (including the skin under the nails). African-Americans and Asians are more likely to develop this form of melanoma.

Nodular Melanoma (This is the type of melanoma I was diagnosed with)

This type is a dome-shaped bump that can appear anywhere on the body. It can be black, dark brown, red or blue, and can have a shiny or scaly texture. These growths quickly *penetrate the body and have the lowest cure rates. 10% to 15% of all melanomas are nodular.*

ABCDE Rule of Melanoma

This is a great way to remember what melanoma can look like and how to recognize the need for a medical opinion.

A = Asymmetric: The mole will **not** be symmetrical. Moles typically are a circle shape with each side basically mirroring the other. Melanoma generally will have one side that has an odd shape compared to the other side.

B = Border: As mentioned above, Melanoma will typically have jagged or uneven edges.

C = Colour: Most regular moles are all one colour. Melanomas can have various shades of brown, black, white, and blue.

D = Diameter: Melanoma tends to be a little larger, although this is not always the case.

E = Evolving: Watch for changes, new mole or a spot that doesn't heal. You won't always see this letter (E) on Melanoma information, but it's important. This is how I recognized mine.

Now, I do have to say here that this is a good general guideline, but you will notice that I have used the words "typically" and "generally" above and that is because my Melanoma did not have any typical signs other than it was "new." It had apparently been there for quite some time, but had evolved and the growth protruded to the outer layer of the skin, which is how I noticed.

Even my doctor did not think it was suspicious. Be very aware of your body and aware of any changes. We are all going to get moles and age spots, but if you listen, your body will tell you when something is off. If you keep looking at a mole or have a feeling about it, simply have it checked. When I was in California for boot camp I would consistently wake up with my hand covering the mole on my butt. It was my body's way of letting me know it needed some help.

THE FOLLOWING FACTORS CAN INFLUENCE THE RISK FOR MELANOMA:

- **Moles** – having a lot of moles

- **Sun exposure** – Excessive exposure can increase your risk. Sun exposure is a major risk especially now that you can burn so quickly

- **Ethnic origin** – As mentioned in the stats above, your ethnic background can be a contributing factor

- **Heredity** – About 20% of Melanoma diagnosis is hereditary. If a relative has been diagnosed, be extra careful and get checked regularly

In 2008, a Melanoma Staging study was completed by the American Joint Committee on Cancer. 60,000 patients participated and results show 5 and 10-year survival rates for Melanoma patients. Percentages ranged from 40% - 97% based on the stage of the cancer. My diagnosis was Stage IIA, so it's a 5-year rate of survival at 81% and 10-year survival at 67%.

My diagnosis was caught early. I have passed the 5-year mark now and look forward to being part of the 67% when I hit 10 years. I consider myself one of the lucky ones. Melanoma can be deadly in a very short period of time.

Our world has drastically changed over the past 30 years and the sun is so much stronger. Protecting your skin is the first step in preventing skin cancer. Please understand the seriousness, especially if you are born after 1990. 1 in 6 chances of developing Melanoma is scary! Think of your closest six friends who like to hang out at the beach and get a great tan. Based on this statistic from the Canadian Skin Cancer Foundation, it means one of you could be diagnosed with Melanoma and could die within months.

Your illness does not define you, your strength and courage does.

UNKNOWN

Chapter 3

Surgery, Recovery, and Results

This chapter will take you through the surgery and reality of what happens when you are diagnosed with Melanoma. It's not pretty, but it's real.

My mole before the removal was simply a new little bump just like you'd see anywhere on your body. It wasn't ugly, or bleeding. It was just simply, new. Being aware of your body and any change that may appear is the first step to early detection.

My mole after the initial removal for biopsy.

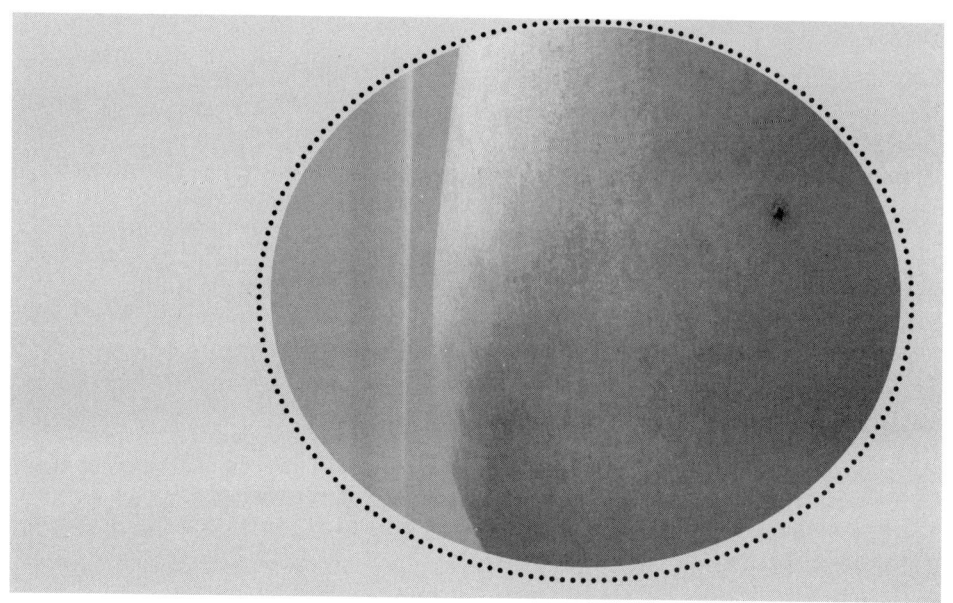

Surgery Day

I sent this e-mail to family and friends just before I left for the hospital

---

November 9th, 2009

Hi Everyone!

Just getting ready to leave for the hospital. A few more hours and it will be all over. YAY!

Have a great day. Enjoy the sunshine (supposed to be nicer than Sunday!) And I will talk to you later.

Keep Smiling :)

Love ya!

Patsy

P.S. Please send me lots of positive and healing energy at 11:00am. Not that I need it, but hey, why not? LOL

Reading this e-mail now with all the exclamation points and positive vibes seems like maybe I was a little more nervous than I let on. I am a very strong woman, but now looking back I think sometimes it was easier to be strong and powerful rather than process what I was truly feeling. I was scared, alone, and vulnerable. These are all tough words for me to associate with myself. I've spent many years telling the world how strong and independent I am. It was cancer that gave me the gift to admit to myself, it's okay to let others in.

I was ready to get the surgery over and done with, so I put on my iPod and started walking up University Avenue toward Princess Margaret Hospital. No one was with me, but as I said, I have always been very independent and truly believe what will be will be. Walking is very therapeutic for me. It's a time for me to take things in and clear my head, so, it seemed like the right way to start my day.

I'm so lucky to have such amazing people in my life. My friend, Sandy was meeting me at the hospital to be there with me all day. She drove to the hospital, but I didn't want a ride. I think it was a chance for me to be a bit defiant. I was strong and I wanted to walk!

As I approached Princess Margaret hospital the song, "The Climb" by Miley Cyrus started playing on my iPod. I got goose bumps just listening to it. I felt a surge of strength.

Here are a few lines:

The struggle I'm facing
The chances I'm taking
Sometimes might knock me down
But, no I'm not breaking
I may not know it
But these are the moments that
I'm gonna remember most
Yeah, just gotta keep going
And I, I gotta be strong
Just keep pushing on

This song has become a sign of strength for me. It has come on the radio or my iPod at other times when I've needed a reminder of my inner strength.

Later that day I sent out another email to my friends and family after surgery.

....

Hi Everyone!

OUCH! OUCH! OUCH! LOL I'm home and feeling great! I walked out of the hospital slowly, but I was walking. YAY! Figured it would hurt more to "sit" in a wheelchair! Everything went really well. I was joking with the staff when I woke up in recovery. LOL!

I don't think they knew how to take me at first. LOL

The staff everywhere in that hospital is simply outstanding. I felt so taken care of all day :) BUT I did take the morphine. Thank God! Butt still hurts, so they gave me OxyContin.

So, I may be still feeling those effects. We'll see how I feel later :)

Doctor was very pleased, and said everything went extremely well and he felt everything looked great. Only had to remove 1 lymph node, so that's got to be good! The doctor said no work this week :(and no physical exercise for 6 weeks.

Holy $%^$^%$$$%^

Anyway, I did promise him that I wouldn't teach boot camp!

Petra and Sandy are staying here tonight and telling me that I don't even look like I had anything done :)

Having a glass of sparkling apple cider with the girls. Champagne substitute for me while they enjoy their wine.

Hope you all got out and enjoyed that beautiful sunshine this weekend and today!

Thanks for all your support through my little adventure :)
Talk soon!

Patsy

The small little bump earlier turned into a
very large covering. The whole cheek of my butt!

I have the most incredible friends, family, clients and boss. I received so many flowers, and e-mail messages filled with beautiful words of strength and healing. That's the only thing that brought tears to my eyes during this entire experience. I definitely felt the love.

I was off for a week to let my body heal properly, but I was very happy to go back

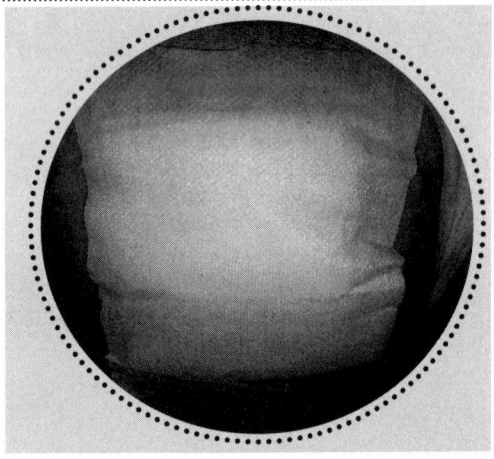

to work! I knew it was crucial to give my body downtime, but sitting at home doing nothing was quite boring for someone who has always been a workaholic.

Yes, I will admit that now, but would have never acknowledged that prior to diagnosis. Do you see why I consider cancer a gift? I have learned so much about health, my deeper feelings, and myself during this process. It's been such an incredible growth period for me. I still probably work too much, but each year I'm getting a little better at adding healing techniques to my lifestyle.

Two weeks after my surgery my bottom looked like the following pictures. Melanoma is not a simple little removal of a mole. Any diagnosis of melanoma will require a wide excision to remove the surrounding tissue so Doctors can test for metastasis (spreading to other areas of the body)

Starting to heal...

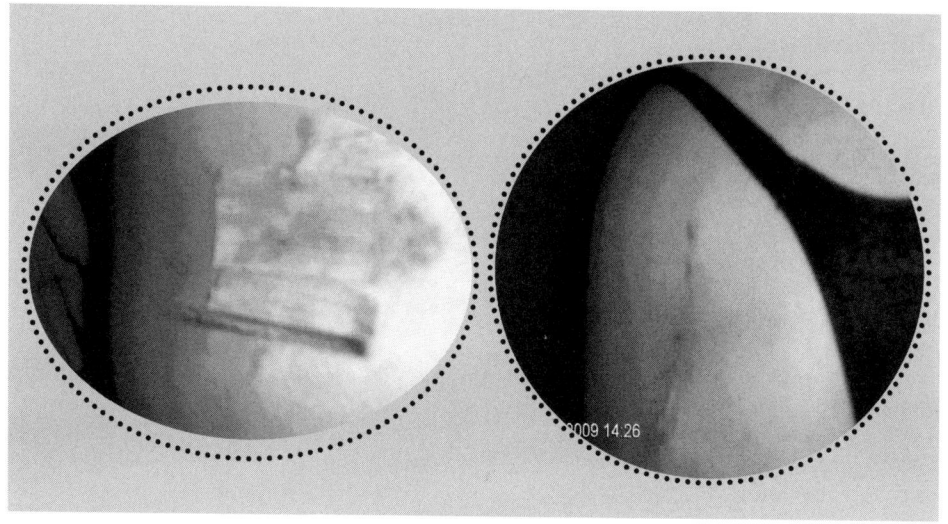

Two weeks after shows the scar and swelling from the lymph-node removal site. The doctor told me it was normal to have a bump there so I thought everything was healing nicely.

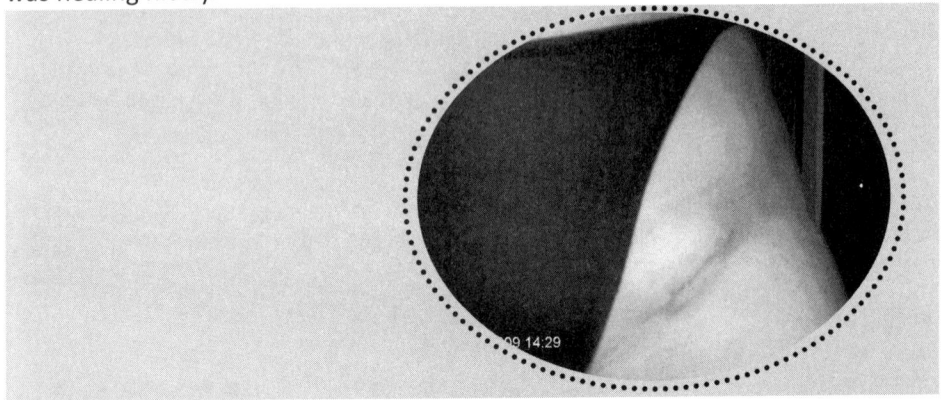

November 24, 2009, Results Day!

Hi Everyone!!

Well, great news! I got my results back today and we got it early :)

Cancer is gone!

Lymph-nodes are clear!

So, on with life... Follow-ups every two months and that's it! Now on to that war against tanning salons and toxins! And to achieve my goal to share all that I've learned about cancer and prevention!

Have a great evening.

I know I certainly will :)

Thanks sooooo much for all your support during the past couple of months.

Still Smiling :)

Patsy

I smiled from ear to ear when I got home. The two months had been a whirlwind and it seemed like a lifetime had passed since I accepted the cruise ship job. I had learned so much about melanoma, toxins and had also grown significantly as a person in such a short period of time. I was very content now to stay right where I was: surrounded by wonderful family, friends and colleagues.

AS IT TURNED OUT, IT WASN'T COMPLETELY OVER JUST YET...

On November 25, 2009, just 1 day after I took the picture of my groin area (above), I woke up at 3:00am and my left leg was on fire. It was red from my thigh to my hip, looked a bit like a bad sunburn, and it was really hot. I was wide-awake, unsure what this could mean and not really wanting to consider that it could be from the lymph-node site. This was pure denial. Looking back, it was obvious that it had something to do with the surgery. At 5am I called Tele-health who said I needed to see a doctor within 4 hours. My struggle between denial (it can't be anything, I'm healthy) and fear (what if the cancer has spread) was a big one. I laid on the couch for another hour, not moving until I could call Sandra at 6am. I knew she would know what to do. When I told her what was happening, her first response was call 911, but I just didn't want to acknowledge it.

Sandra hopped in her car and drove from Barrie to take me to the hospital. She truly is my rock. Unfortunately, by the time she arrived, nausea and weakness had set in and I was unable to stand. She had to get a wheelchair from my concierge, which was a tough dose of reality for me.

After several hours at emergency, they determined I had a bad infection in the lymph-node removal site. The swelling in my groin area wasn't normal after all. The doctor on-call drained it and sent me home with antibiotics.

Two days later, my Dad was undergoing heart surgery at Newmarket hospital, so I drove up in the morning still in some pain, but I wanted to be there. When I met Sandra there she was concerned that I was still limping (she's a Mom). She said the antibiotics should be working by now, so we went to the washroom so she could look at it. She was not impressed and thought the infection was spreading. After my Dad went into the operating room, we went down to the emergency room to have it checked out.

The doctor took one look at it and asked for my antibiotics. Within a couple of minutes I was hooked up to an IV antibiotic and he was on the phone to my doctor in Toronto to tell them I would be coming in.

My Dad came out of surgery and was doing great. So after I gave him a kiss, I left to drive back to the city with the IV in my hand. Somehow I knew I needed to park my car at home as this was not going to be a short hospital visit. At Mount Sinai hospital, with Sandra by my side, they did a proper draining of the site. In the words of my sister, "Oh My God, there was buckets of pus oozing out."

I'm glad it was her watching and not me! I'm surprised I didn't break her hand, I was squeezing it so hard. This was so painful! Tears were involved. So that definitely means it was on the high end of my pain threshold.

They kept me in the hospital for five days as it was that serious. Apparently I could have died. The infection was called Cellulitis, which started in the lymph-node removal site and it spread very quickly. The wound was so deep from the infection that they were packing it with gauze strips two times daily, and the skin tissues inside were so raw they were giving me morphine to combat the pain.

Just because I was afraid of what it could be, I ignored some unusual signs like swelling in the groin area and I delayed medical attention in a very serious situation.

When family and friends came to visit me in the hospital during my recovery, I could see the concern on their faces. I was terribly weak, hooked up to poles and after a cancer diagnosis people do tend to think the worst. I could have prevented all this by just listening to my body. It was giving me the signs that it needed some help, but fear kept me from responding.

Now I've found a definition for fear. False Experience Appearing Real.

I remind myself of this when fear shows up in my life and creates a negative scenario in my head.

During my hospital stay the nurses were great, but the food left a lot to be desired. Preserved, packaged, phony food heated in microwave ovens. Seriously? People in hospitals are sick and should be receiving the best nutrition possible to help the body heal, not garbage full of toxins! I swore off their food after 2 days and my sister brought me real food. This is something that needs to change.

December 2, 2009, Home

My home nursing was two times a day for another week and then once a day for a month. Yes, you read that right, *One month*. I had two amazing male nurses who alternated each night to pack the wound. They were like my new committed relationship. All I did was work and come home to my nurse. I had to go to a clinic in Barrie everyday during the Christmas holidays to have the wound packed while I visited my family there. It was crazy how much nursing was required to bring me back to full health.

Finally, I parted ways with my nursing team. It was so great to have my life back to normal. I missed my regular routine and just enjoying life! I was back to exercising which was awesome. It had been four months since I had really worked out consistently or completed a long run. It was time to change that. I signed up to run the Chicago half-marathon in July. My friend, Jill, and her son Kayden, came to cheer me on for my first attempt at running 13.1 miles again.

This was more than just a race.

This would mean I was back.

The run was going along perfectly until mile 7. At this point, I started to feel mild pain in my infection site. Nothing really bad, just something felt like it was rubbing together inside my hip and groin area. It was a mental run from that point on and then around mile 9 when my struggle was getting worse and I honestly wasn't sure if I could finish. My iPod started playing The Climb, by Miley Cyrus, which is the same song I listened to during my walk to Princess Margaret on my surgery day. Tears welled up in my eyes and I thought, "I can do this, I've been through so much. This is nothing."

I replayed that song for four miles, and right up until the finish line with a respectable time of 2 hours, 11 minutes. Not my best time in numbers, but certainly my best race for accomplishment. I was back! I went on to run Disney half-marathon in 2 hours, 7 minutes and I haven't stopped since.

After a couple months back at work, I was offered and accepted a new job as Director of Group Exercise at the club. I thought I had to change jobs to make a full-time career in fitness and management. This was yet another lesson given to me from this whole experience. Let life happen. Sometimes we try so hard to make things happen the way we think it should be. What's meant to be will be. If you just work hard and believe in yourself, life will give you everything you need.

After cancer and the infection, I look at my body so differently now. It truly is an incredible human machine. My body has overcome cancer and a life-threatening infection. I'm so proud to say that. Yes, I had medical help, but after five years since surgery, my body is in great health without any reoccurrence. I treat my body with great respect now, as I believe cancer does not just happen randomly. There are many controllable contributing factors. I thought I was very healthy at the time of diagnosis. I ate well, exercised daily, and looked great. I have since realized that looking healthy does not actually mean you are healthy. There is so much more involved in staying healthy in our toxic world. I had some pretty obvious contributing factors.

There are moments when the human body can overcome things you would never expect.

ANDRES INIESTA

CHAPTER 4

BUT I WAS SO HEALTHY. HOW COULD THIS HAPPEN TO ME?

My description of cancer and what is "healthy" have changed drastically within five years. Like many, I thought cancer was something that happened to other people, not healthy people like me. Anyone can develop cancer. Yes, even the "healthiest looking" people.

WHAT IS CANCER?

After reading several books by experts in the field, this is my interpretation:

Cancer is the result of stress, nutritional deficiencies and a compromised immune system. The body is out of balance in some area and disease is a symptom of a bigger picture of your overall health. Balance incorporates a healthy mind, body, and spirit. When your body is in balance in all three areas it is, "at ease", when it's out of balance it's "dis-ease." This is how I look at any change in my body. I look for the imbalance.

People may argue that their hereditary factor passed down cancer, and I don't dispute there can be a connection. Could it be that in a lot of cases the hereditary factor is that family members have developed similar habits and food choices? If there is a strong hereditary factor, then it is even more important to continually support your immune system to help it keep disease away. Our body's immune system must be compromised in order for cancer to grow. We all have cancer cells, in my case damaged DNA from a bad sunburn. As you read on, you will see the deficiencies and imbalances within my body that led to cancer.

WHY DO SOME PEOPLE GET CANCER AND OTHERS DON'T?

Nutrition, exercise, and emotions all affect the immune system. All of these functions affect your stress levels, which will then inevitably affect your immune system leaving you vulnerable for disease.

We can no longer look at cancer the way we did 30 years ago. It is not a disease that picks you. Unfortunately, we now live in a world with many toxins that are beyond our control and a healthcare system that is financially tied to treatment rather than prevention.

In the book, "How you can beat the killer diseases", Harold W. Harper, M.D. and Michael L. Culbert state:

What if cancer is a systemic, chronic, metabolic disease of which lumps and bumps constitute only symptoms? Will this not mean that billions of dollars have been misspent and that the basic premises on which cancer treatment and research are grounded are wrong? Of course it will, and in decades to come a perplexed future generation will look back in amazement on how current medicine approached cancer with the cobalt machine, the surgical knife, and the introduction of poisons into the system and wonder if such brutality really occurred.

I believe the body knows how to heal itself if given the proper tools but there are situations when surgery, chemo and radiation treatments are beneficial. I know a few people who have had some or all of these treatments for high stage cancers and have survived several years, but all of them have incorporated a very healthy diet and lifestyle changes with a strong focus on highly nutritious foods (predominantly plant-based) and limited processing. The sad part was that they all discovered this by reading and researching. Not one of their doctors suggested making the dietary changes they have made.

Now, in their defence, doctors are only required to study approximately 25 hours of nutrition in Medical School, so can we really expect them to know?

Doctors learn to successfully identify and treat the symptoms they are presented. First, we need to learn for ourselves how to prevent symptoms from developing and eliminate the need for cutting, burning, or poisoning ourselves in order to get better.

I know that sounds harsh, but it really is what we're doing. We all need a healthcare team consisting of a Medical Doctor and a Naturopathic Doctor. It's a winning combination.

The body is made up of the mind, body and spirit. If treated as a whole unit, it will thrive. Surgery, chemo, radiation may remove the existing tumour, but if the underlying problem is not addressed, *will the cancer come back?* Sure it will. But you can help your body prevent that from happening by bringing all systems into balance.

Listen to your body. It will tell you all you need to know.

After my diagnosis and months of research I discovered just how many toxins surround us daily. It is imperative that we keep the immune system strong by avoiding these toxins as much as possible.

Our world of affluence has done us a great disservice. Think of all the luxuries we take for granted. What are they really doing to us? Are we really the fortunate ones?

Life Luxury:	_Toxins:_
Machines, Cars, Trucks, Indoor, Recycled Air, Mass Production	Air Pollution, germs, lack of fresh oxygen Air, ground, and water pollution _Tips To Reduce:_ Avoid idling vehicles, areas of high factory output, heed environmental warnings such as air quality and beach restrictions Get out and enjoy nature! Plants give us oxygen so try to spend time around grass, trees, flowers Buy some indoor plants
Life Luxury: X-rays, Airport Scanners	_Toxins:_ Radiation _Tips To Reduce:_ Avoid X-rays for minor aches and pains Request a pat-down instead of walking through the scanner. It's your right to request it and reduce your exposure.

Life Luxury:	Toxins:
Computers, Cell Phones, Television	Electromagnetic Radiation from technology
	Tips To Reduce:
	Turn off electronics when not in use. Remove all TVs, computers, phones from your bedroom to ensure a sound night sleep

Life Luxury:	Toxins:
Alcohol	In*toxic*ation. Intoxication is derived from a Latin word meaning "to poison"
	Tips To Reduce:
	Limit alcohol to special occasions, not a daily indulgence

Life Luxury:	Toxins:
Bottled Water	Plastic leaching into water, landfill leaching into ground
	Tips To Reduce:
	Purchase a high quality water bottle to keep with you. This will not only reduce plastic build-up in the landfill, but will encourage you to drink water consistently throughout the day.

Life Luxury: Restaurants	*Toxins:* High fats, excessive sugar and salt, low quality foods *Tips To Reduce:* Make restaurant meals a special occasion. You will avoid excessive toxins and appreciate the experience when it's not a daily routine
Life Luxury: Mass Food Production	*Toxins:* Pesticides, hormones, genetically modified organisms, animal cruelty *Tips To Reduce:* Know the source for the foods you buy Discounted food doesn't equal healthy choices and could result in you paying with your health
Life Luxury: Boxed, packaged convenient foods	*Toxins:* Preservatives, food colouring *Tips To Reduce:* Prepare and purchase fresh food from nature to avoid these unnecessary additives

Life Luxury:	Toxins:
Vitamins, Drugs	Man-made synthetic, foreign chemicals that our bodies don't recognize
	Tips To Reduce:
	Not all vitamins and drugs are made the same
	The drug industry is worth a lot of money and fillers are cheap. Ask your HealthCare professional to recommend what they would give their children
Life Luxury:	*Toxins:*
Coffee available on every corner	Consume excessive caffeine, sugars, processed chemicals, artificial additives
	Tips To Reduce:
	Drink good quality coffee or tea without all the extras. Some lattes have hundreds of calories and also contain ingredients full of chemicals.

100% Ban against tanning beds in Brazil

100% Ban against tanning beds in Australia planned for 2015

Several US states, Canadian provinces, and European Countries have all placed a ban for anyone under 18

CENTERS FOR DISEASE CONTROL AND PREVENTION

THE CONTRIBUTING FACTORS IN MY CANCER DIAGNOSIS ARE AS FOLLOWS:

Tanning Beds

I used a tanning bed, but it was never a regular occurrence. It was more in my late twenties and early thirties when I thought looks were so important. I can't believe they can still be in business.

The World Health Organization has added tanning beds to the Class #1 list of cancer causing substances, which is the same category as cigarettes, harmful chemicals and X-ray radiation.

The cumulative damage or 1 bad burn caused by UV radiation can lead to premature skin aging (wrinkles, lax skin, brown spots and more), as well as, skin cancer.

In Oct 2013, Australia announced its plan to join Brazil on a complete ban of all commercial tanning beds effective 2015. Other countries such as United Kingdom, France, Germany, Austria, Belgium, Finland, Italy, Norway, Portugal, Spain, Sweden, Northern Ireland, Scotland, Wales, Iceland, some Canadian provinces, and some U.S. states all implemented some form of protection. This can include a ban on indoor tanning for teens under the age of 18, or a warning label right on the bed.

According to the FDA, one required label would read, "Persons repeatedly exposed to UV radiation should be regularly evaluated for skin cancer."

Hopefully more countries will move towards a complete ban in the future.

Australia has the highest skin cancer rate in the world with an annual diagnosis in excess of 300,000 people from a highly preventable disease.

Research shows that over 80% of all new cases of cancer in Australia are skin cancer.

Research also shows that regular use of tanning beds under the age of 30 increases risk of melanoma by 75%. Almost a guarantee that anyone under the age of 30 using a bed will have skin damage potentially leading to melanoma. Scary.

Sun-Tanning

Did I love the sun? Absolutely! I can't deny that. I used to go on vacation a few times every year and came back with, what I thought, was a fabulous tan.

A tan, whether you get it on the beach or in a bed is not healthy. Tans are caused by harmful ultraviolet (UV) radiation from the sun or tanning beds, so if you have a tan you have sustained skin cell damage. Yes, we all need Vitamin D and studies show 10-30 minutes a day can allow your body to produce sufficient amounts. Everyone's tolerance is different, so be careful not to burn your skin.

Winter months create a problem for those of us living in the northern hemisphere so supplementation is required. There are excellent supplements that a Doctor or Naturopath can recommend based on your individual vitamin D test results. This is a simple blood test that can be done to show if deficiency is an issue, and it is for many people. Good idea to have it checked. Studies indicate Vitamin D deficiency is extremely important in disease prevention.

Vitamin D is extremely important, but our environment has changed so much that skin burns within minutes of being exposed without protection.

I had never paid attention to what the news reports were saying about UV. In fact, I didn't even know how UV rays worked. I was just always too busy to pay attention. Do you know the difference between UV rays? How we are continually damaging this process by daily habits? I thought it would be good to review.

The Sun and your Skin

Ozone Depletion Process:

The Ozone layer is a thin shield around the earth that protects us from harmful UV rays and makes life possible here on earth. Our advances in technology, manufacturing, and luxurious living are some of the sources that slowly deplete this protective layer. Unless we make some changes to our environment, things will only get worse. The comforts of our life such as the fridge, freezer, air conditioning, cars, planes, fireplaces, manufacturing plants, aerosol spray, and cow off-gassing of methane all release toxins into the atmosphere and contribute to this situation.

As this protective layer thins, UV rays will be stronger here on earth. UV rays are the cause of non-melanoma skin cancer and play a huge role in Malignant Melanoma. UV rays also contribute to Cataracts, a disease of the eye's lens. It's definitely a very different world than it was 30 years ago. I remember being able to sit outside for hours without getting burned, now, it's a matter of minutes.

ULTRAVIOLET RAYS

UVA	HEALTH CONCERNS:
- Penetrates into the deeper layers of the skin (Epidermis and Dermis layers), very damaging to new skin layers - Constantly present, all season and weather - Penetrate clouds, clothing, glass windows - Tanning beds primarily emit UVA, potentially 12 times stronger than the sun. - If under the age of 30, tanning beds increase skin cancer risk by 75%	Premature aging, suppressed immune system, sun spots, leathery skin, wrinkles, Cancer
UVB - Penetrates into superficial skin layer (Epidermis) - Stronger in summer months between 11-3pm - Reflects off snow, water, sand, concrete - Need to protect skin all year round	**Health Concerns:** Sunburn, Cancer
UVC - Doesn't penetrate Earth's surface	

SUN PROTECTION FACTOR Number, what percentage of protection does it offer?

SPF 15 = 92%

SPF 30 = 97%

SPF 40 = 97.5%

As you can see the percentage increase becomes minimal above 30 and a concern with high SPF numbers is people can feel a false sense of security staying out in the sun longer without reapplying. I generally just like to be covered with clothing, but any exposed areas I use a 30 SPF and keep reapplying.

A lot of people have sustained damage from tanning salons and the sun, so why hasn't everyone developed skin cancer? A great analogy I read from the China Study by T. Colin Campbell, PhD and Thomas M. Campbell II, MD

"THINK OF CANCER LIKE GRASS SEED. IF THE SEED DOESN'T HAVE THE RIGHT CONDITIONS OF WATER, SUNLIGHT AND NUTRIENTS, IT WON'T GROW. IT'S THE SAME WITH CANCER."

ALCOHOL

Enjoying a couple of drinks a day (mostly rye and diet coke) and a few extra on weekends was not uncommon during my twenties, thirties, and early forties. Little did I know what I was actually drinking...

DIET COKE, ASPARTAME

There are many side effects and independent research indicating the health risks of aspartame. An article from Brian Clement of Hippocrates Health Institute identifies that when the temperature of aspartame exceeds 86°F, the wood alcohol within it converts to formaldehyde and then formic acid (the poison found in the sting of fire ants). This may contribute to metabolic acidosis, creating excessive amounts of acid. Potentially compromising kidney function. He also notes that aspartame is a neurotoxin and "can cause a plague of neurological diseases, changes the dopamine level of the brain, goes past the blood brain barrier and deteriorates the neurons of the brain."

Anything that's potentially messing with my brain is banned from my life. Unfortunately, it's very hard to get definitive information as the diet health world is worth a lot of money. Government agencies continually defend it and say it's safe at certain levels. I believe aspartame is very bad for the body and a contributing factor in my weakened immune system. Coke and Pepsi have recently agreed to reduce the levels of the caramel artificial food colouring in soft drinks after the Consumer Reports Food Safety & Sustainability Center warned of a link to cancer in the news.

RYE

Overconsumption of alcohol will tax the immune system and the liver, which is one of the key organs responsible for cleaning the body.

Once alcohol is ingested, alcohol enters the stomach where approximately 20% is absorbed immediately through the stomach into the bloodstream. The rest then passes through to the small intestine and into the bloodstream where it stays until it can be metabolized, and broken down by the liver. The liver can only process ½-1oz of alcohol per hour so if you drink more, the alcohol simply accumulates in the blood and travels around the body. Remember the Latin meaning for intoxication? To Poison.

So when I was drinking excessively, I was essentially poisoning my body every day.

These are just a few organs that can be negatively affected by alcohol: Liver, Brain, Heart, Pancreas, and compromising your immune system, which we know leaves you vulnerable for life-threatening disease. I drank regularly and usually excessively on weekends for 20 years. I'm not surprised at all that I developed cancer. My body was so under-nourished and running on toxic overload.

Cleaning the body is a crucial part of health and removing toxins. The liver is an intricate part of cancer prevention as it removes harmful toxins from the blood and helps detoxify the body. Several experts have made the connection and claim that when cancer is diagnosed you can be assured that the liver is not functioning at its maximum capability. The good news is that the liver is the organ that can regenerate! You can assist your liver by eating enzyme-rich foods like raw vegetables and fruits, and eliminate drinking alcohol.

The **colon** removes waste. Your food choices have a huge impact on this process. When you are constipated, back-up occurs and poisons remain in the intestines. These toxins are absorbed back into the bloodstream causing the liver to work harder to clean the body. Constipation itself should be considered a serious disease, as it is a precursor for so many preventable diseases. It's very disturbing to know that some people don't seem too concerned and find it acceptable to have a few bowel movements per week.

The body is an incredible machine, and if one of these systems breaks down, it will naturally transfer extra work onto the other systems.

Cancer needs a compromised immune system that is brought on by unhealthy lifestyle choices.

Tanning was my "seed" and alcohol, stress, and nutritional deficiencies were the water, sunlight and nutrients it needed to grow. Stress and nutrition control are so instrumental that each topic warrants its own chapter.

In general, we can say that the blood is only as clean as the bowel.

BERNARD JENSEN, D.C.

AUTHOR OF TISSUE CLEANSING THROUGH BOWEL MANAGEMENT

Chapter 5

Stress – A Silent Killer

"Wellness is an active process of becoming aware of and making choices toward a healthy and fulfilling life....A state of complete physical, mental, and social well-being, and not merely the absence of disease or infirmity."

The World Health Organization

Yes, stress is a silent killer. Stress is now an accepted daily reaction in life, but that's not what it's supposed to be. The body's stress response is a physical biological response that happens to protect us from danger, not because the line-up is too long at our favourite coffee shop. You've seen that person, who's upset, stressed, constantly checking his or her watch, and tapping the toe. Imagine what's happening to the body while this is going on, and all because the coffee wasn't served immediately.

Road rage is another example of a stress reaction out of context. When the body is stressed it triggers the release of our fight or flight hormone to protect us from danger. Some of the physical reactions are a faster heartbeat, increased blood pressure, faster breathing, muscles tightening, and increased senses preparing us to fight or run away.

Stress is not a necessary response to a coffee line or a traffic jam. Stress is toxic when it's a regular occurrence and there are many times we don't even realize we're stressed. We can recognize it in others, but not always in ourselves.

Life is so fast now and full of deadlines, frustrations, challenging relationships, demands of children, divorce, and financial struggles so taking "down time" can seem out of the question. Stress is the deciding factor between staying healthy or developing life-threatening disease and early death.

Stress is identified in two ways, external and internal. My own experience shows external stress was caused by hidden internal stress. Thoughts and emotions are involved in everything we do. We all have stress in our lives, but it is how we deal with it that affects the body. Work was a huge "unrecognized" stress factor for me, as I always took on more than I needed. Being busy meant success in my world, but after my diagnosis I realized it was also a crutch to cover up what was happening internally.

Most people have a "crutch" at some point in their life and feelings that aren't acknowledged. If you're not busy, does that mean you're not successful? If you're not out socializing every night, does that mean you're not popular? If you're not in a relationship, does that mean you're unlovable? We put a lot of pressure on ourselves to be something other people or society wants us to be instead of just being who we are.

For me, my need to be so good at my job was due to an insecurity of "not being good enough". Because I didn't properly address this feeling, the external stress of my career and strong need to succeed was really a reflection of my internal fear of failure. This fear carried over into my relationships, pushing people away to protect myself against rejection. I didn't recognize any of this back then, but I now know these were strong signs of internal stress, suppressed feelings and a breeding ground for disease.

Internal stress is sometimes the most difficult type of stress to understand or acknowledge. However, it is the most **important** and can be an underlying cause of many diseases. This is not to suggest that physical disease isn't real, just that the physical symptoms represent only part of a bigger picture. The body is complete when mind, body, spirit are balanced.

Work:

Work is probably the biggest stressor for most people. There will always be deadlines, commitments and authority figures. Some days may be more intense with higher expectations, but learning to prioritize effectively is the key. Turn your "To Do" list into 3 categories:

1) Must do today

2) Should do if possible

3) Could do if time permits

Just breaking up your list into these categories will reduce the overwhelming feeling of having too much on your plate. Always being busy isn't always a sign of too much work, it can simply be more about organizing, prioritizing or making changes where necessary.

Learning that it's okay to say no is an essential way of honoring yourself. This is really important to me now, as I want to have the time available to say yes to the special people in my life.

Family should be #1, but mine was not for many years. Work trumped everything and I also felt stress from the guilt of not being available. Since my diagnosis, I know work will always be there, but making time for family and friends is a key to reducing stress.

Relaxing and laughing reduces stress instantly. Many of us have a balance issue between work and life. If we think back just 30 years ago, life was very different. Families generally always had meals and evenings together, weekends were for family and friends, remember those leisurely days wondering "What should we do today?"

What happened to those days? Needing to succeed in business became such a huge priority so we could buy all the expensive material things to prove our worth in society. Relationships changed, communication changed and now we have a world full of negativity, judgement, insecurity, sickness and high stress. There's a connection.

I lived this way for many years making career my number one focus. Although I haven't let go completely yet, I'm making huge changes that are moving me very quickly toward my goal to live a much simpler life surrounded by positive family and friends.

Physical Aches and pains happen to everyone the odd time, especially now with the addition of so much technology. Physical stress can be a result of sitting at a desk or computer too long. Movement is a huge factor in keeping the body healthy and stress-free as we will learn later in the book. I was lucky to be involved in competitive sports from an early age that developed a love of exercise that has kept me active and fit all my life. Exercise was the one thing I was doing right in my lifestyle, that helped prevent some of the other side effects of sitting at a desk for 14 hours a day. Since my diagnosis, I have continued to exercise, but I also incorporate regular walks in nature or by water everyday to clear my mind and quiet my body. Even if it's just a walk in a park with some deep breathing, the benefits are numerous, such as a calm mind, healthy body, inhaling oxygen that feed the cells, and a break from the mind's continuous thoughts. We live in a beautiful world, but I think sometimes we overlook the very things that feed our soul.

I'm going to ask that you open your mind in this section as this information was very important in my journey and is crucial in my healing. I believe my cancer diagnosis was due to sun damage, toxins and withholding anger and feelings. The mind/

body connection is an essential part of staying healthy. Emotions are normal and an important part of life, but when an emotion becomes excessive or suppressed, it becomes a threat to the health of your body.

During the past 5 years I've learned a lot about the mind/body connection and Traditional Chinese Medicine (TCM) shows how this connection can manifest in illness. This holistic approach to health has been practiced for thousands of years. It brings balance and harmony to the body/organs via our energy flow.

Acupuncture is a technique used to free any blockages in the energy flow by inserting small needles along specific points in the body. Tongue and pulse analysis, herbal medicine, massage, nutrition and exercise are additional ways Chinese Medicine is used to create balance within the body. It's fascinating how the body responds to simple techniques.

According to TCM each organ is associated with a specific emotion and suppressed feelings can create disease and compromise the function of the associated organ.

Below is a table that identifies the specific emotion that is attached to each organ based on Chinese Medicine.

Emotion	Related organ
Anger	Liver/Gallbladder
Joy	Heart
Worry/Pensiveness	Spleen
Grief/Sadness	Lung
Fear	Kidney

Due to circumstances and life experiences, I learned to take care of myself at a very young age. Externally, I did that very well, but internally I was a bit of a mess.

Unfortunately, I didn't realize it. Living on my own from the age of 18 was challenging. With limited guidance, I learned to count on myself and control all areas of my life. Managing a full-time job, night school, and attending a lot of parties always kept me busy and I never really had to deal with my emotions.

I had some long-term relationships, but they were never deeply emotional for me as I never let my guard down. My life was great on the outside, proving to others that I could do anything on my own, rarely asking anyone for help. I will admit, it's still very hard for me to ask for assistance, but I recognize it now as my fear of appearing weak. I believe this is true for many people.

Looking back, I know I had buried some pretty strong feelings of loss, anger and rejection for a very long time. Everyone in my life thought I was doing amazing and that I was so accomplished. Everyone, except me. Oh, I knew I was successful. My material things proved that, but I never really felt good enough in all areas of my life.

I was a perfectionist, due to fears and distrust. We all have a story of our past, some a little more difficult than others, but in the end it comes down to how we process these stories and the emotions attached to them. Holding on to the past can create disease in the body, as it did in mine.

Hanging onto things and mulling over "what if" or "if only I had" leads to suppressed emotions, internal stress and potential disease.

In my case I never shared what I was feeling and was unable to release the anger. Well, you will recall from my introduction that I had my Gallbladder removed in my twenties. It's pretty young to have that kind of surgery. If you look at the Chinese Medicine Chart above, was it completely surprising?

No. I think it was clearly a sign of ill health and ill-emotion. Years later, those feelings were still unresolved and my liver was quite obviously stressed emotionally as well. With the addition of my unhealthy lifestyle of consuming alcohol, unhealthy foods, and prolonged hours of sitting, I'm not at all surprised that a serious disease was in my future. You may even know someone who was diagnosed with cancer and you were so surprised because that person looks so "healthy." Healthy looking doesn't always mean healthy in all areas of life. Do *you* look in the mirror and see complete health… mind, body and spirit?

Emotional healing begins with acknowledgement. Just like we have "gut feelings" on decisions, we also have intuition on aches and pains in our body. If we just listen carefully, we'll know what the body needs. Emotions are part of being whole and if we shut down or suppress them we're not functioning as a whole unit. I try very hard now to say what I'm feeling and yes, even things others don't want to hear. It's all in the delivery. People will get over it and I will let it go. It's so important to my future health.

EMOTIONAL BALANCE

Here are 5 great ways to help bring your body back into balance:

1) Meditation/Mindfulness

Taking a break during your day to quiet the mind will have incredible effects on your overall health.

I've been meditating regularly now for a few years and I can honestly say it has changed my life. Meditation is different things to different people. There is no right or wrong way of doing it. Some people go much deeper into their meditation, but I believe any amount of time spent meditating or quietly reflecting can work wonders on your body. There are several guided meditations online that you can listen to. Begin with guided mediation, as it will allow you to experience the peace that can be yours simply by closing your eyes, listening to a soothing voice with the sounds of birds or a waterfall in the background.

2) Walk in nature

When was the last time you went for a quiet walk in nature and just enjoyed the surroundings? I know, it's difficult to justify the time when you have so much to do. Allow yourself 15 minutes to sit quietly in a park, stroll by the water or trees, or lay on the ground and find images in the clouds. Remember doing that as a kid? Take a moment to really notice the beauty that surrounds you. This will do wonders for your overall well-being.

I had a very stressful day this summer. I was at a conference until 2:30pm then had to quickly go home to change and be on the highway by 3:00pm to drive up north as there was a baseball game ending, and if I was any later I would be sitting in traffic. I made it onto the highway by 3:00pm, but was still on a deadline to arrive up north in time for a surprise 80th birthday celebration for my Mom. With about 30 minutes left in my drive I started to have some light discomfort on my left side just under my ribs. I had never experienced this before and calmed myself by doing some deep breathing as I drove. It was scary, but I knew my body was trying to tell me something. I arrived at my sisters and said, "I need your bed and 15 minutes". She asked why and I said I don't know what's wrong, but I know I need to meditate. I spent 15 minutes with a healing meditation and the pain was gone. I'm not kidding!

We made the surprise party on time and had a wonderful evening. Instead of rushing back to the city the next morning as I had planned, I stayed up north and we went for a walk by the lake. I listened to my body. It needed nature. I took off my shoes, walked barefoot in the grass, dangled my feet in the lake and enjoyed the sunshine.

The pain was a strong sign that I was, once again, taking on too much and allowing stress to be a regular part of my day. Stress is never going to go away completely, but it's how you respond to it that matters in the healing process. The Spleen is on the left side, just under the ribs where I was having the pains, emotionally attached to worry in the Chinese medicine chart, not surprising. Since this episode I have continued to ensure I limit stress. The pain has never returned.

3) Yoga

Just like meditation, yoga can have an incredible effect on your health. The combination of calming music and focus for the mind, movement for the body and a calming feeling for the spirit, results in a complete healing environment. Yoga has many different styles and can incorporate incredible strength, relaxation and gentle movements, which are all beneficial both mentally and physically.

Life can be crazy and stressful, but with the incorporation of a yoga practice, things just won't seem so stressful and important, at least not for a little while. Not to discount the importance of work deadlines or family/social commitments, but it's about the balance, *your balance*, and the time for you is just as important as those other things.

There is a calmness that comes over me when I enter a yoga class. My body relaxes, thoughts from the day go away as I am absorbed in the positive energy of the environment and the soothing voice of the instructor. Ending my day with yoga helps put the day's events, negative or positive, into perspective.

Self-awareness and inner guidance will lead you to balance....you just need to listen.

PATSY MCLEAN

4) Tai Chi and Gi-gong

Tai Chi and Gi-gong are gentle mind-body movement exercises based on the energy flow in the body. Energy is called chi or qi. This energy flows through meridian lines (energy pathways) and in Chinese Medicine it is believed that a blockage in the qi can cause illness in the body. Specific movements create a healthy flow of energy. This is a very calming, meditative movement that can be done anywhere in a short period of time to relieve stress. This practice is quite new to me. I haven't found a local class to attend yet, so I just put on a YouTube video in the comfort of my home for 10-30 minutes and know that I'm assisting the energy flow of my body.

5) Deep Breathing

Deep breathing exercises will contribute to a much more productive day. Did you know deep breathing is a great way to invite more oxygen into your cells? There is a connection between sitting for long hours and reduced oxygen levels in the cells. Deep breathing is a simple way to increase oxygen and energy flow to avoid potential illness. When you take a deep breath your abdomen should expand, not just your chest.

Close your eyes, take a long, slow deep breath, hold for a couple of seconds and then slowly release, push all the air out so you empty your lungs completely.

Complete 5 full breaths and then resume your work. You can practice this a few times a day standing or sitting. You will feel the difference.

6) Reiki

Reiki is a Japanese healing technique administered by a Reiki Practitioner via hands to help balance the energy of the body. Reiki promotes well-being in all areas of the body including emotions, mind, body and spirit. Energy blockages can contribute to illness and Reiki can help release these blockages. Anything we can do to keep the energy flowing will promote a healthy balance. I am now certified as a level 1 Reiki practitioner and plan to continue my studies in this area as energy flow is so important in disease prevention.

THE IMPORTANCE OF SLEEP:

Stress can play a huge role in how well you sleep and vice versa.

Sleep is the time when the body works on repair and detoxification. If your sleep patterns are out of balance then your health can become compromised. Studies have shown that those who sleep less than 6 hours per night consistently can have a shorter life expectancy. Sleep has an incredible effect on our mental, emotional and physical well-being.

Your body has a big job at night helping detoxify and repair cells from the daily load of toxins. Lack of sleep can affect your immune system, hormone balance, and overall health. Think of sleep as the time your body is tidying up any negative energy from the day so you can be at your best the next day.

Does lack of sleep contribute to weight gain?

Lack of sleep can cause a disruption of the Neuro Endocrine System. We have two hormones that regulate our food intake and lack of sleep can cause an imbalance in this area.

1) **Leptin** is released from fat cells to let us know we've had enough to eat.

2) **Ghrelin** is released from the lining of the stomach to tell us when we're hungry.

Now, if you don't get enough sleep and these hormones become unbalanced, then the body can become confused, getting the wrong signal, at the wrong time, and potentially resulting in weight gain.

SYMPTOMS OF SLEEP DEPRIVATION:

- Physical exhaustion

- Difficulty sleeping or excessive sleeping

- Poor concentration and decreased productivity/motivation

- Irritability and moodiness

- Lack of creativity
- Low tolerance for stress
- Regular colds or infections
- Indecision
- Weight gain

What happens when you sleep?

There are two main sleep categories with a series of stages, which are crucial to the health of your body and mind, non-REM and REM.

Non-REM (Rapid Eye Movement):

Within Non-REM there are 3 stages the body goes through:

N1 (Transition to Sleep):

This stage is approximately 5 minutes in length and is the time your body slows down. Eyes still move slowly under the eyelid. You will still wake up quickly in this stage.

N2 (Light Sleep):

In this stage you are actually asleep for approximately 10-25 minutes. Heart rate slows, eyes stop moving and there is a decrease in body temperature.

N3 and N4 (Deep Sleep):

This is the real sleep stage. You are sleeping, however your body is now going to work.

Welcome to the repair and detoxification stage. This is a crucial time for your body, so if you limit the amount of time it has in this stage, you are not allowing the body to do an important job. If you don't sleep deeply enough or long enough, what do you expect to happen to the repair of your cells? Continual deprivation can potentially lead to

diseases such as diabetes, heart disease, compromised immune system, and high blood

Insomnia is your body telling you something is out of balance. It's time to listen...

PATSY MCLEAN

pressure to name a few. This phase is crucial to restore the physical energy required to keep the body healthy.

REM (Rapid Eye Movement) Sleep:

This is the dreaming stage.

What can you do to improve sleep quality?

- Exercise during the day or at least 3 hours before going to sleep.
- Avoid caffeine, alcohol, chocolate, sugar, spicy foods, or a big meal close to bedtime.
- Enjoy some time in nature. Get some fresh air. It's always a huge benefit especially if you work indoors with artificial lighting.
- Regulate your sleep schedule. Go to bed at the same time to regulate sleep patterns. Read something light so your mind has time to calm.
- Ensure your bedroom is free of EMF's! (Electro Magnetic Frequency) Yes, Television, cellphone, and computers can affect how well you sleep.
- Your bedroom should be quiet and dark, so your body will know it's time to produce Melatonin, the sleep hormone.
- Yoga, meditation, and deep breathing are all excellent ways to calm the mind and body allowing it to fall into a wonderful, peaceful sleep.

Stress was a huge factor in my life for years, but it wasn't the visual stress that is usually associated with the word stress. This was stress from my own internal dialogue and high expectations of myself to always prove my worth. I was very successful in business as I went above and beyond the expectations of the client so they would always be happy with my work.

Now, that may sound like good business practices, but not if it comes at the expense of a balanced life.

I was career driven to a fault. Burying myself in work to avoid dealing with feelings of loss and insecurity I had experienced in my personal life. I always judged others who couldn't handle career expectations and long hours or cried for days over a relationship breakup. To me that seemed "weak" and unproductive.

Now, I know judging others was the easy way to not deal with my own deeper feelings. Being "strong" ironically was a huge contributor to my illnesses.

It was hard to admit or acknowledge but I now believe most cancers are brought upon ourselves by several "lifestyle" habits, stress, and emotions. I know mine are pretty obvious when I look back on the lifestyle I was living. "The good life" took its toll and withholding unresolved feelings topped it all off.

The sorrow which has no vent in tears may make other organs weep.

Henry Maudsley

As I shared earlier, I learned early to bury my feelings and put on the happy face no matter what I faced. Unfortunately, without releasing those feelings, disease can and did develop (a couple of times).

Although there are a lot of "environmental" contributors to cancer, I believe stress management, food, and exercise are the 3 most important things we can control to help prevent cancer from starting or growing. Yes, in my case, the sun was the initial culprit, but if I'd known then what I know now, it would never have developed into cancer. But, this was my gift. My journey.

I was indeed blessed to know Dr. Selene Wilkinson as her response to my diagnosis was much different than is typical in the medical field. Not discounting the advances medicine has made, but I've known several people now who have been diagnosed and not told of any food changes they could make to assist the body.

The recommendations I've heard about are always we can "try" Chemo or radiation. Why not "try" changing the Standard American/Canadian Diet too? There is significant research that shows cancer thrives on high sugar, excessive animal proteins and a toxic environment from chemicals and preservatives in packaged foods. So why don't doctors recommend adjustments to diet and lifestyle? I know this will change in the future as more doctors become aware of the nutritional factors contributing to cancer. Patients have the right to know what changes they can make to assist their body. The perfect combination will be when we see medical and naturopathic doctors working together to heal patients.

Selene's reaction, "there is so much we can do" gave me a different way of viewing cancer. She gave me hope that cancer didn't have to mean a time limit on my life. Selene was the teacher that I needed at a crucial time in my life and I am so grateful for the gift she gave me. Her gift to me was faith. It was faith that if I learned how nutrition affects the body and how toxins can cause havoc within the cells I could assist my body to heal during this process.

When cancer is diagnosed, most people aren't this lucky. They are usually directed right into surgery, chemo, radiation, and follow-up drugs never understanding the need to support the body and help it heal. I will be forever grateful that I have the privilege to know Selene and continually learn from her. She is one amazing lady.

We all have cancer cells, but if our immune system stays strong, it can prevent cancer cells from ever mutating and attacking the body.

We have daily toxins present in our environment that can weaken our immune system if not countered by strengthening the immune system. Think of how much more you can do physically if your muscles are strong. Your immune system is the same. If given the proper tools to keep it strong, the white blood cells will work hard to eliminate any foreign toxins and keep you healthy!

Dr. Wheeler stated in her book "The Conquest of Cancer":

"The ability of your immune system to successfully prevent cancer is directly dependant on your state of nutrition."

Convenience = Cancer!

Patsy McLean

Chapter 6

Digestion and Elimination

The body is amazing and knows exactly what to do to keep us healthy and vibrant if given the proper tools. Before my diagnosis I did not understand the complexity of my body and how all systems worked to process what I ingested. I thought I did, but it was a real eye-opener when I started to see how negatively my choices were affecting my body. If your body is not digesting food or eliminating toxins properly your body will be stressed leading to a compromised immune system and potential disease.

How can we assist in the digestion process?

1. Eat healthy real enzyme rich food that has nutrients for the body to easily absorb. Raw vegetables and foods cooked under 115°F come with their own enzymes putting less stress on the body.

2. Drink lots of water! Water makes up 70% of the body.

   Did you know?

   Brain = 75% water

   Blood = 92% water

   Bones = 22% water

   Muscles = 75% water

   In addition, water is required to regulate our body temperature, carry nutrients and oxygen to cells, help convert food, help absorb nutrients, remove waste, breathe, and protect organs. Water has a very important job!

   Stats show a large part of the population walk around mildly dehydrated on a regular basis. Here are some signs you may need to increase your water intake:

- Thirst
- Dry skin
- Dark/coloured urine
- Dry mouth
- Fatigue/weakness
- Chills

3. Avoid or limit alcohol consumption

    Remember what we learned in chapter 4? The liver can only metabolize ½-1oz of alcohol per hour and any excess simply accumulates in the blood and body tissues until it can be processed. The Latin meaning for *intoxication* is *to poison*.

    I drank regularly and usually excessively on weekends for 20 years. I'm not surprised at all that I developed cancer. My body was so under-nourished and running on toxic overload. I'm so thankful that I learned.

4. If you haven't yet, stop smoking.

    There are negative effects of smoking on all body systems, not only digestion.

5. Exercise! Keeping the body in motion will assist all systems to work more efficiently.

6. Eat slowly, chew food completely, and eat smaller quantities.

    This will allow your body to process the foods. Large quantities of food in one sitting add extra stress to the system. Take your time, relax and let your body do its job.

7. Reduce stress

    As we learned in Chapter #5, stress is really hard on the body, but trying to break down food while the body is dealing with other issues puts extra strain on the entire body.

8. Listen to your body

    It will tell you what foods work for you and what foods don't. A simple example for this is gluten. A lot of people get very bloated after consuming products containing gluten. Your body is telling you it can't process it, so why ask it to?

    Allergies to certain foods can cause skin reactions or swelling. Again, your body is giving you key information. Learning what foods assist *your* body to work at an optimal level is crucial to great health.

ELIMINATION:

Digestion is imperative to give the body the nutrients it needs, but our elimination processes are just as important. There will always be toxins in our body from the world we live in so all the elimination systems of the body must be working optimally to remove them. Let's look at the main elimination systems:

Colon: This is your main sewer system in the body. The Colon removes all waste from anything not converted to fuel for the body.

Lungs: Remove carbon dioxide. It's crucial that we are expelling all those inhaled toxins

Skin: Your skin is your largest organ and toxins are removed via sweat. Very important. Skin eruptions can indicate a buildup of toxins that don't have a way out. Check your skin so you recognize if there is anything new or changed.

Lymph: Transports waste from your cells to the blood stream so the liver and kidneys can do their job to filter the blood.

Kidneys: Filter the blood and remove toxic waste.

Liver: Although not considered an "elimination" organ, it is very important in preventing disease. The liver has to work hard to process every toxin that comes into the body. The more you feed it, the more overworked it's going to be, leading to a compromised immune system. This happened to me. Between food and alcohol my poor liver must have been working overtime everyday.

If one of these systems is overworked and not functioning properly it puts more stress on all the others leading to potential disease.

How can you help your organs?

Colon: Eat food from nature

Lots of organic vegetables and fresh juice will definitely help keep your sewer clean.

Lungs: Exercise, deep breathing, meditation, and yoga.

Anything that helps you breathe deeply and calmly.

Skin: Dry brushing

Removes dead cells and toxins along with stimulating to encourage cell renewal.

Lymph: Move

Walk, exercise, skin brushing, or a mini-trampoline called a rebounder. Just 10-20 minutes jumping up and down is a great exercise to assist the body. The lymph system does not have a pump like the heart muscle, so movement helps it work. Since the job of the lymph system is to transport waste it is crucial that it keeps moving so there is no stagnation.

Kidneys: Drink water

How much do you need? An easy calculation is 50% of your body weight. (Eg. 130lbs = 65 oz. or eight 8 oz. glasses per day.) More exercise will increase your requirement.

Liver: Eat healthy food and reduce alcohol

Garlic, ginger, turmeric, beets, carrots, green leafy vegetables, green tea and avocado.

I must mention **Lemon Water.** This is an incredible tool in the quest for great health. Squeeze half a real organic lemon in warm water to start each day and your entire body will thank you. It helps cleanse the body and keeps it functioning optimally! Just remember to use a straw to eliminate any tooth damage from the citrus or rinse your mouth with coconut oil to neutralize acid from the citrus.

ACID AND ALKALINE:

You've probably heard the term PH balance as it is a common phrase in the health world. It's not new but how to keep the body alkaline is now referred to regularly in magazines and on the Internet.

Let's determine what PH Balance really means:

PH means Potential Hydrogen, and is the acidic/alkaline level in a solution. In this case, the solution I'm referring to is your blood. The acid/alkaline balance scale is 0 - 14. 0 - 7 is Acidic and 7 - 14 is Alkaline. The human blood PH level is 7.35 to 7.45. What you ingest determines how hard your body has to work at maintaining that number.

Over the long term, too many acidic foods can put additional stress on the body systems and disease can develop. Just think how much extra energy your body is using to keep this balance if your diet is predominantly acidic on a regular basis. This is very common in today's world.

When your body is working harder to maintain the PH level, another area of the body may be compromised. Balance in all areas of the body is key to optimal health. Our society is so busy now that most people think "food on the go" is a necessity, but most of that food is processed and acid forming.

I was a perfect example of being too busy to prepare food. I do believe **Convenience = Cancer** and this is how our world now lives, hence the increase in so many horrible illnesses. People are "tricked" by great marketing into thinking they're eating healthy foods. There is a lot of money to be made in the food industry when they use less than desirable products, but make them look fresh and healthy.

Stress negatively affects our body chemistry in so many ways, including the PH balance in the blood. So if you are highly stressed, eating food on the go, and not committing to regular exercise and deep breathing, you are a perfect candidate for disease.

Chapter 7

Food Comparisons – Then and Now

The food you eat can be either the safest and most powerful form of medicine or the slowest form of poison

– Ann Wigmore

I am sharing what has worked for me over the past five years and the research I have done that brought me to these conclusions. Everyone should do their own research to discover what's right for your body as there are a lot of hidden factors in our food today that shocked me when I discovered them. If I can help just one person, then my book has been a success. I'm still learning every day and discovering new things.

This will be a life-long journey as new information and research is updated.

When I was diagnosed with cancer and Dr. Selene Wilkinson gave me my "Cancer Food Protocol" it unleashed a very strong "need to know" feeling in me. I started researching **everything** only to find that what I thought was pretty healthy eating was, in fact, actually contributing to the growth of my cancer.

On the next page is a chart showing the foods that I ate almost daily prior to diagnosis. High protein meat and low carbs to keep you lean, strong and healthy…..or so I thought. I've also identified whether the foods are acidic or alkaline in the body.

These foods seemed very healthy, but yet still convenient with my hectic schedule. I didn't have hours to spend preparing food, so paying a little more to have it prepared for me made sense.

Little did I know that the price I would pay would be my health…

The ability of your immune system to successfully prevent cancer is directly dependant on your state of nutrition.

VIRGINIA LIVINGSTONE-WHEELER,
THE CONQUEST OF CANCER

Healthy Looking, Isn't Always Healthy

Breakfast Options	Acid/Alkaline
Coffee	Acid
3 Boiled Eggs	Acid
Whey Isolate Protein Shake	Acid
Raspberries/ Blueberries Apples/ Banana	Acid
Whole Wheat toast with Peanut Butter	Acid
Bacon & Eggs	Acid
Quick Oatmeal	Acid

Lunch/ Dinner/Snacks	Acid/Alkaline
Whey Isolate Protein Shake	Acid
Chicken/Cheese	Acid
Rotisserie Chicken/Salad	Acid/ Alkaline Combo
Turkey Wrap	Acid
Egg Salad Wrap	Acid
Wild rice with chicken and veggies	Acid/ Alkaline Combo
Fish and Salad	Acid/Alkaline Combo
Protein bar/Snack	Acid
Apple with Peanut Butter	Acid
Microwave Popcorn	Acid
Chips/Week-end treat	Acid

Reviewing the foods I had been eating was quite shocking to me after I had learned about the acid/alkaline chart. These foods look pretty healthy, right? It's not that some of these foods aren't healthy, it's just the quantity of acidic foods I was eating and the imbalance that created in my body.

We need a balance of approximately 80% Alkaline and 20% Acid to keep the PH balance. As you can see, the majority of my nutrition was on the Acid side, which is the case for a lot of people. The Standard American (and Canadian) Diet is typically 80% Acid and 20% Alkaline, exactly the opposite of what it should be for optimal health.

How I used to eat doesn't look unhealthy, but it was definitely nutritionally deficient due to the limited variety. I practically lived on eggs and rotisserie chicken. Always removing the skin so it was healthy? Not so much, since those chickens can be injected with fat, sugar, salt, flavourings, etc.

It's not a bargain for your health if you can buy a prepared chicken for 5 bucks. There may be more "quality chickens" available now, but my body is very happy eating a high alkaline diet with no meat. Remember, **Convenience = Cancer.**

My body was working overtime to maintain the critical PH balance in my blood. Combine that with the stressful life I was leading and it was a recipe for disaster. Does this sound like you? Many people are still living this life, hence the increase in cancer and disease. You can change this and avoid becoming a statistic. Our bodies give us little clues to the state of our health. Listen to your body...exhaustion, irritability, those little aches and pains all mean something.

Try doing a chart of your food, for your own knowledge and to see if there are areas you can improve. You can view a great acid/alkaline chart at www.energizeforlife.com to determine if you're eating a good balance.

SPECIAL "ACIDIC" CONSIDERATION – CANCER LIKES SUGAR

Sugar is acidic in the body and there is more and more information identifying the dangers of sugar. You may have read some of the articles or books that have been in the news over the past year about how detrimental sugar is to our health. Contributing to obesity, diabetes, heart disease, and the big one...cancer. There are a lot of reports stating sugar feeds cancer and others that dispute this theory. It makes sense to me that sugar impacts our health and increases the potential to develop disease.

According to Don Ayer, Ph.D., a Huntsman Cancer Investigator and professor in the Department of Oncological Sciences at the University of Utah:

"It's been known since 1923 that tumor cells use a lot more glucose than normal cells. Our research helps show how this process takes place, and how it might be stopped to control tumor growth."

When I was researching sugar I also discovered this information on the Positron Emission Tomography (PET) scan that is commonly used to detect cancer growth.

This test is frequently used to determine if cancer has spread to another part of the body. The patient is injected with a simple sugar called FDG "Fluorodeoxyglucose". This scan works as **cancerous tissue uses more glucose than normal body tissues**. Tumor sites light up during the PET scan so doctors can see where the cancer is located. The more glucose the cells take up, the more the cells light up, confirming where the tumour is. Does this prove sugar could contribute to cancer growth? I believe so. As a cancer survivor, it just makes sense to me that I would want to limit my sugar intake…..it's my health. It's so important to do your research and make your own opinion when it comes to your health.

MAIN FOODS ON MY CANCER PROTOCOL:

Breakfast Options	Acid/Alkaline
Daily Juice Carrot Celery Dandelion Root Burdock Root	Alkaline

Nut Cereal Almonds Cashews Brazil Sunflower seeds Flax seeds Organic apple juice	Acid/Alkaline Combo
Wheatgrass	Alkaline

Lunch/ Dinner/Snacks	**Acid/Alkaline**
Daily Soup Garlic Wakame Seaweed Shiitake Mushrooms Burdock Root Leeks Beans or grains Onion Turmeric Root	Alkaline
Green and Root Vegetables	Alkaline

Below is a table showing how these foods, along with specific supplements helped me correct the damage I had done to my body. I've included the benefits column to show how we were detoxifying my body and feeding it immune boosting foods. I did not waver from this list.

FOOD CHOICES AND SUPPLEMENTS IMPORTANT BENEFITS

Sun Chlorella (Cracked Cell Chlorella)	
Single celled fresh water algae renowned for its amazing nutrient content and health benefits. Chlorella is a whole food and a complete protein. Includes all 20 Amino Acids including a great balance of the eight essential Amino acids. Rich in vitamins, minerals, and highest chlorophyll content of any plant. SUN Chlorella is grown in Indonesia and manufactured in Japan. It's the highest quality I have found. Beware of some brands that have been grown in Japan with potential nuclear implications. Do your research.	**Chlorella helps** - Detoxify the body of harmful toxins while still nourishing it - Stimulate the immune system - Promote growth and healing - Help repair the body at a cellular level while potentially promoting anti-cancer activity - Help the body utilize oxygen and purify the blood - Eliminate toxins all while nourishing the body - Increases the antioxidant glutathione levels in the body - Binds and eliminates toxins like heavy metals, pesticides, artificial food additives/preservatives, etc

Daily Soup Ingredients and Benefits:	**My thoughts:**
Garlic: General immune stimulant **Wakame Seaweed:** Helps bowel inflammation, contains B12 and Iodine **Shiitake Mushrooms:** Boost immune system and believed to stop or reduce tumours **Burdock Root:** Controls blood sugar, antibacterial, antifungal and desmutagenic (inactivate mutagens/cancer causing agents), high fibre and source of potassium	As you can see all the ingredients in the soup had a general theme of boosting the immune system and fighting disease. I also included some other vegetables and beans in the soup for variety and additional nutrients, but these were the consistent ingredients. I still often make this soup, especially when the colder weather arrives and lots of people are suffering from colds and flus. It never hurts to boost the immune system.
Daily Juice Ingredients and Benefits:	**My thoughts:**
Carrot: Antioxidant, anticancer, boosts immune system, antibacterial **Celery:** Anticancer, diuretic **Beets:** Antibacterial, antioxidant, cleansing **Dandelion root:** Supports liver, gallbladder, kidney, and bladder **Burdock Root:** Controls blood sugar, antibacterial, antifungal and desmutagenic (inactivate mutagens/cancer causing agents), high fibre and source of potassium	My protocol had me drinking a small glass of this juice 4 times daily. When you read the benefits you can see why. Once again, the theme is improving the immune system, supporting vital organs and reducing cancer-causing agents. I have included information about the benefits of juicing in the juice recipe section.

Wheatgrass: 2 oz. of wheatgrass is equivalent to approximately 5lbs of raw organic vegetables giving you therapeutic amounts of nutrients to support the immune system. It's also a wonderful detoxifier for the body, especially the liver and blood. It also helps detoxify the body of heavy metals, and toxins stored in the body. Definitely an important addition to anyone fighting disease. At Hippocrates Health Institute, Wheatgrass is incorporated into the raw food diet 3 times per day	**My thoughts:** *Ann Wigmore is an Icon who healed herself of cancer by eating wheatgrass and herbs. I recommend you read her story. Ann co-founded the Hippocrates Health Institute and became the driving force behind the alternative health movement for more than 25 years. Such a great story.* Note: You can buy wheatgrass 'flash-frozen" to keep in your freezer. It looks like an ice-cube tray and you simply pop a couple in a glass, let them melt and voila…you have your morning wheatgrass shot. Wheatgrass is also available in a powder form
EAT A VEGETARIAN DIET ONLY **THESE ARE THE EXACT WORDS ON MY CANCER PROTOCOL.**	**My thoughts:** There are a lot of "vegetarian" controversies and negative comments, but it has changed my life. Changing my diet from high acidic meat consumption to a high alkaline vegetarian diet saved my life. Doing your own research and not listening to others isn't always easy, but you must make your own decision and choices when it comes to your health.
Protein Source: Grind Almonds, cashews, brazil, sunflower and flax seeds Add 2 tbsp organic apple juice, mix and let ferment overnight in the freezer Morning: add hot water and it's a warm cereal full of nutrition	**My thoughts:** So many people ask vegetarians about protein sources. This is a great one. There are many others that I share in the recipe section

Supplements:	**My thoughts:**
Selenium: cancer preventative B12 & folic acid: turns off oncogenes, a gene that has potential to turn cancerous Vitamin C: cancer preventative Vitamin E: cancer preventative Zinc: boost immune system and cancer prevention Bromelain tablets: Interferes with Malignant growth	Everything on my cancer protocol was boosting my immune system and allowing my body to heal. These supplements were loading my body with cancer prevention.

As you can see, this was a huge change from my previous food chart. Was this a difficult change? Yes, it was but probably not for the reasons you're thinking. Selene's words stuck in my head "There is so much we can do". This wasn't about being deprived from eating the foods I used to eat...it was about saving my life...and learning new ways of living. The hardest part for me was the shopping and finding out where to buy all these new foods and supplements. Selene directed me to an organic grocery store called The Big Carrot in Toronto. I had never shopped there before and now it's my favourite store.

I continued on this protocol for a full year from diagnosis. The next step for me was understanding that I could incorporate other foods back into my life without the fear of a reoccurrence. That has definitely taken some time and has been the hardest to process. For me it was all or nothing, so being handed a sheet with what to eat was much easier than having too many options. The gift of learning continued as I learned how to cook and prepare delicious foods on my own.

Two years after my surgery I learned about **Hippocrates Health Institute**, an outstanding raw food facility in West Palm Beach, Florida. This institute has helped many people make the dietary changes to assist their body with healing naturally. After receiving traditional treatments and given a limited time to live, the results from the lifestyle changes were astonishing. I had the good fortune to spend a week with Brian Clement, Ana Maria Clement, both directors at the institute, and 70 others either fighting cancer, in remission, or learning to prevent cancer.

The experience was unforgettable. I didn't know what to expect when I signed up for the one-week retreat other than it would be raw food, seminars, and blood tests to determine health. I ate only raw food, consisting of mainly salads, for a week leading up to the retreat so my body would be somewhat prepared. I was shocked when I started to discover all the amazing "raw food" options that were at each meal. Pasta from zucchini noodles, Taco's from nuts and spices…the list goes on and on. Chef Ken was amazing and each day we were lucky to spend an hour with him learning how to prepare the food. It was fascinating to me. I've included some of my favourite raw food recipes in the recipe section.

I learned and felt the benefits of a raw food diet during the week. I had lots of energy, completely satisfied, and loved all the flavour that comes from great spices. We also had outstanding daily seminars and presentations from experts including renowned medical doctors who had been in practice for 30+ years. These doctors recognized that something wasn't working in the medical field and had combined naturopathy in their practices. The topics ranged from cancer prevention, the effects of hormones, benefits of infrared saunas, meditation, vitamins, new technology and so much more. Naturopathic and conventional medicine working together is a combination we need in our world to prevent and reduce disease.

During the week I spoke with people who had stage 4 cancers years earlier but with the help of Hippocrates they were able to make the necessary lifestyle changes and reverse the cancer growth. Yes, reverse cancer growth. Talking with these people who had maintained their health for many years after a diagnosis of months to live brought tears to my eyes. These people were real and very thankful to be alive. It was like they had been given a new life and a new body.

I spent time with a lady who had completed conventional treatments, but the cancer had returned. After her second treatment, she was not given much hope. This is when she learned about the Hippocrates Life Change 3-Week Program. In this program she learned how nutrition, exercise and mindfulness play such a huge role in health.

When I met her at the retreat she had been cancer-free for seven years and was continuing to thrive by fueling her body with healthy nutrition, exercising daily and living calmly. She came to the retreat to renew her passion and remind herself of the importance of her choices to reduce stress with yoga/meditation, take time to prepare nutritious food, make time for daily exercise, and enjoy life with family and friends. She knew that ultimately these choices make the difference between cancer-free and reoccurrence. She shared with me that it had been difficult sticking to nutritious meals when her family preferred traditional meals like meat and potatoes, while she was trying to maintain a plant-based healing lifestyle. It's not easy to stay committed when there is temptation all around us.

The result of these common lifestyle changes for most of the people I met was that they were truly living their life in a very balanced way...not just existing or overworked...like so many people. The stories were all very similar. Diagnosed with high stage cancer, after or without treatment, they enrolled in the program at Hippocrates and learned to live a lifestyle incorporating raw food, exercise, and stress management/calming techniques. The one- week Malibu retreat that I attended was a beautiful experience and a perfect confirmation for me that everything I was learning and living would keep me healthy for a long time. I'm continually working on stress management, and it continues to get better each day.

It has taken five years and I am much more relaxed when making my food choices as I have so much more knowledge. I still maintain a no meat lifestyle as it works well for my body and I believe high animal protein does contribute to disease. I have incorporated more variety as you will see below in my **current food chart** below.

Breakfast Options	Benefits	Acid/Alkaline
Lemon Water (1/2 fresh organic lemon squeezed in warm water)	Boost immune system, balance PH level, stimulate digestion/help absorb nutrients, help metabolize fat, clear skin, cleanse lymphatic system	Alkaline (Although lemon appears acidic, it is alkaline in the body)
Matcha or Green Tea	High level of antioxidants, boost immune system, benefits over-all health protecting against disease	Alkaline
Green Rooibos Tea	Rooibos tea is Caffeine-free and hydrating, antioxidant, high mineral content, good for circulation	Alkaline

Green Drink (spinach/celery/ turmeric root/ burdock root/ spirulina or sea vegetables (algae)/ ginger/hemp seeds	Green veggies are loaded with vitamins, minerals, fibre, and natural enzymes that play a crucial role in digestion. Great for immune system and removing toxins from the body	Alkaline
Sunwarrior protein powder Plant based protein made from brown rice	I use this supplement when I feel I need to increase my protein for muscle building and repair. This is the protein supplement recommended by Dr. Brian Clement, Hippocrates.	Alkaline
Selene's Nut Breakfast Almonds, cashews, brazil nuts, sunflower and flax seeds, grind, mix with 2 tbsp organic apple sauce, freeze overnight. Add hot water in the morning for a tasty cereal	High protein source and vitamins/ minerals including Vitamin C, Selenium, Healthy fats	Acid/Alkaline combo

Quinoa Organic berries Nuts Buckwheat Flax/Chia or Hemp Seeds Any combination of the above is a great source of nutrients	Complete protein, source of fibre, iron, calcium, potassium, magnesium Antioxidant to help boost immune system and detoxify, healthy fats, vitamins, minerals	Acid/Alkaline combo
Organic Steel Cut Oatmeal Organic berries Nuts/Seeds Cinnamon Hot cereal on a cold morning.	Protein source with antioxidants for immune system, healthy fats, fibre vitamins, minerals	Acid/Alkaline combo

Holy Crap Breakfast Cereal Yes, this is really the name! This is an awesome store-bought cereal, convenient and healthy Buckwheat, chia, hemp, raisins, cranberries, apple bits and cinnamon. Also a version without the fruit/sugars called Skinny B	Buckwheat has been called the World's Healthiest Food. Full array of nutrients, protein, fibre, carbs, vitamins, minerals, and good fats	Acid/Alkaline combo

Lunch/Dinner Options	Benefits	Acid/Alkaline
Salad and vegetables	Organic vegetables provide vitamins, minerals, fibre, and natural enzymes for digestion. Boost immune system and detoxifies the body	Alkaline

Quinoa with vegetables	Complete protein, high caliber carb, fibre, iron, calcium, potassium, magnesium Boost immune system and detoxifies the body	Alkaline
Sprouts (Alfalfa, Fenugreek, Mung Bean, Sunflower)	High protein source	Alkaline
Buckwheat Pasta This is not wheat. Buckwheat is a fruit seed from the Rhubarb family	Protein source, antioxidant, high fibre, anti-inflammatory Great substitute for cereal, pasta, grains	Alkaline
Green Soup Healthy green veggies blended in my Vitamix until warm.	Loaded with vitamins, minerals, fibre. Great for boosting the immune system	Alkaline
Sweet Potato	High in antioxidant Beta-carotene, source of fibre, vitamins, folate and potassium	Alkaline

Zucchini Pasta	Source of vitamins, minerals	Alkaline
Kelp Noodles Both great as pasta substitute	Kelp is a powerful Algae that contains over 70 nutrients and minerals, great addition to any meal	Alkaline
Spaghetti Squash Pasta	Source of fibre, vitamin A, potassium	Alkaline
Butternut Squash Pasta	Anti-inflammatory, omega 3, beta-carotene	Alkaline
Cauliflower/ Avocado/Garlic "garlic mashed potatoes"	Antioxidant, anti-inflammatory, high fibre, healthy fats	Alkaline
Shiitake or Portabella Mushrooms	Immune support, anti-cancer, anti-inflammatory, antioxidant	Acid

Apple/Almond butter snack	Protein, vitamin C	Acid/Alkaline
Almond butter/ dehydrated flax cracker snack	Protein, healthy fats	Alkaline
Nuts (almonds, sunflower and pumpkin seeds)	Protein, healthy fats	Alkaline

As you can see most of these items are Alkaline. The foods I've identified as acid/alkaline combo contain only a small portion that is acidic. Using these items as my base allows for the addition of some more acidic foods without a concern of throwing the balance off. Remember 80% Alkaline and 20% Acid = Perfect balance.

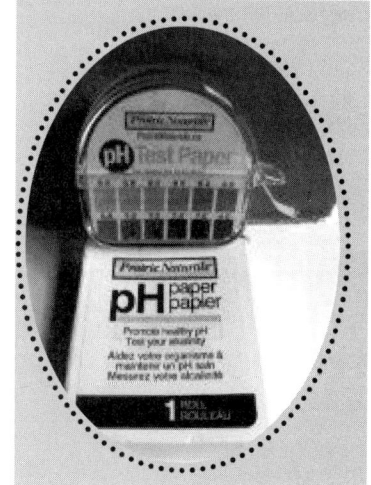

This is a great little tool to check your level, PH Strips.

You can buy them at most health food stores and by putting a little strip in your mouth or in urine (more accurate), it will give you a gage based on the colour it turns. It won't be 100% accurate but will give you a fun way to ensure you are on the right track.

Chapter 9 includes some of my delicious recipes that incorporate many of the foods shown in the chart. Raw food living really can be delish! Is this all I eat? No, these are the main ingredients I choose and if I go to a restaurant I look for the healthiest meal on the menu. Most restaurants now have vegetarian options or a nice salad. I also eat more cooked foods during the winter months as the body does need the warmth. I make a fabulous bean and rice or quinoa soup. Lots of garlic, onions, spices that make it super tasty. I find it the most difficult to find healthy warm food at lunch since I don't use a microwave. There are a couple of "healthier" options near my work, but I do prefer my own meals at home.

As you can see I'm strict, but not completely restricted. It's truly not difficult once you make the changes and feel the difference in your body. When I made the changes Selene suggested, I felt an increase in my energy. I remember being aware of this as someone asked me if cancer made me tired. I thought for a moment and said, "No, I actually have lots of energy."

I think that's when I started to put the pieces together that this new way of eating was fuelling my body in a way it had never been fuelled before. I didn't consume alcohol, caffeine, sugar, meat, or anything the body had to work hard to digest. All it needed was my assistance. Infusing my body with all these nutrients allowed my body to recover from surgery and that horrible infection. I'm sure it would have been much worse if I had fallen back into my old eating habits. The gift of cancer helped me understand the importance of my choices and the impact they have on my health.

I look back on the "convenience" of the food I used to eat and I cringe knowing what I was doing to my body. Food prepared at home tastes a lot better, costs less, and I know what's in it. Convenience was a habit I developed over the years that fit with my hectic lifestyle.

Knowing you're giving your body the best nutrition possible is an awesome feeling. Do I ever indulge? Sure, when I'm out with friends I will have alcohol occasionally, but my drink of choice now is not Rye/Diet Coke (poison). Now I will ask for: Vodka, water, cucumber, mint leaves. I know, some people say that sounds like salad in a glass, but it's actually quite refreshing and from what I've read vodka is the cleanest alcohol you can drink. It's acquired the name "the Patsy" with my friends. I can't drink much anymore as my tolerance is very low, so 1 or 2 drinks is the max on a rare occasion and I feel it.

The toughest part of making some of these changes can be the people around you. My family and friends have always been very supportive, but sometimes I do feel like I'm offending them a little when they've made a beautiful meal, such as turkey and all the fixings at Thanksgiving. I know they put a lot of time and love into preparing the meals, but I choose what I want to offer my body based on what has been working for me over the past 5 years. It's running like a really well-oiled machine so I want to ensure it stays that way.

The main restrictions that I make are sugar, animal protein and processed foods. Research shows that these foods all have an effect on our state of health and the potential for cancer. Removing sugar and processed foods from the diet is a must for anyone facing cancer, but also for all of us who want to support the immune system and not encourage the growth of cancer or any other disease. Animal protein is a personal choice, but do your research and know where it's coming from because not all animals are raised in the same way and you may not be receiving the nutrition you think you are. Also remember that meat is acidic.

There are completed studies like The China Study that directly link high animal protein to cancer in a lab study with rats. They were able to control the growth of cancer in the rats by changing their diet from high protein to low protein. Sure, there's controversy around the book. There always is where cancer is concerned.

There are also numerous amazing stories of people healing their bodies from cancer by changing to a vegetarian or vegan diet. Hippocrates Health Institute has some incredible testimonials on their website from people all over the world. My cancer protocol was also very specific to "Vegetarian only." It's a personal choice, but I definitely recommend doing your own research and having an open mind to the potential dangers of excess animal protein...make up your own mind....it's your body and you have full control over how healthy it is.

SUPPLEMENTS:

Is great food all we need?

Some people may be blessed with an incredible body that is functioning optimally, but for the majority of people I would guess that some supplementation is required. Meeting with a Naturopath is an ideal way to see any particular deficiencies or weaknesses before it becomes a problem. I supplement regularly with the following:

Chlorella	I still take chlorella morning and night to ensure toxins are continually removed from my body (Note: be sure to research Chlorella brands due to potential radioactivity if grown in Japan)
Vitamin D	As I don't spend a lot of time in the sun and live in the northern hemisphere, supplementation is required. I take 4,000 IU in 4 sublingual drops every day to ensure levels are optimal
Vitamin B12	Since my diet is predominately plant based, I supplement 1,000 mcg in a sublingual tablet daily
Vitamin C	Studies show C is important in cancer prevention so I supplement 1,000-2,000 mg daily
Omega 3	Good for cardiovascular, immune and nervous systems. Joints, brain, skin, and hair all love it too! Overall great addition to a healthy lifestyle. I supplement 2 tbsp., and eat a variety of foods high in Omega 3 such as avocado, walnuts, and flax or chia seeds.
Burdock Root Tinture	Burdock Root is desmutagenic, which inactivates mutagens/cancer causing agents, so I supplement with a tincture (30 drops in glass of water and I'm good to go!) if the root is not available. Burdock root is high in fiber and potassium too.

Turmeric Root Tinture	Turmeric is known as a cancer fighter so I also like to incorporate it as often as possible either by adding root or tincture to food and smoothie
Probiotic	It's so important that your gut health is optimal as this is where your body absorbs all its nutrients. It won't matter what great foods you eat if your body is unable to absorb the nutrients!
Deep Immune	If I'm feeling a little tired, am a little stressed, or just feel I need some immune strengthening I'll take Deep Immune to help boost my immune system and give my body some extra help. The main ingredient is Ashwagandha, a very powerful Ayurveda herb considered to increase energy, prevent disease, and strengthen immune system, just to name a few! Of course, that makes sense if your immune system is strong your body will definitely feel optimal, thus preventing illnesses.
Rejuvenate Cell Therapy	Rejuvenates description: *immediately releases oxygen to the body at the cellular level, and the highest quality, natural minerals, enzymes, electrolytes and amino acids are delivered simultaneously throughout the body. Since they are in the most bioavailable and effective form possible, they go to work on the deepest cellular level.*

As you can see from the descriptions, I am constantly assisting my body to process the daily toxins that may enter my body.

As a cancer patient or survivor, it is important to remember that cancer doesn't grow overnight. The body must be in a state of deficiency or the cancer won't grow, remember the grass seed analogy?

Grass won't grow unless it has sun, water and nutrients. Cancer won't grow without the ideal conditions such as an acid environment, compromised immune system, excess sugars, excess animal proteins, and processed food.

In my opinion, this means we need to work even harder and be even more diligent with our diet to ensure the body stays in a state of optimal health to keep the cancer from returning. If you simply go back to the old habits that created the deficiencies, why would you think the cancer wouldn't return? I'm constantly on the alert to what my body is telling me. Not fearfully, just simply aware...

Bowel movements are another very strong indication of your health. It's not a topic most people want to talk about, but it can tell you a lot about what's happening in your body. Some people think its okay to only have a bowel movement every two days.

Think about that. Your colon removes toxic waste from your body. How is allowing waste to stay in your body for two days okay? Optimal health means 1-3 bowel movements per day. Think of it as food in, waste out. Simple.

With the amount of **toxins** in our environment and food this is more important than ever and should not be underestimated. Why? Your intestines are responsible for absorbing nutrients into the body so transition time needs to be regular to prevent any stagnation in the body. The body and all its systems were meant to be used everyday. By the time the food becomes waste it has gone through all your body's processes and the body has decided what nutrients it can use. The rest becomes waste/faecal matter. It also contains other toxins your body is trying to remove. Our food is very different today...

Until we are willing and able to make the connections between what we are eating and what was required to get it on our plate, and how it affects us to buy, serve and eat it, we will be unable to make the connections that will allow us to live wisely and harmoniously on this earth.

Will Tuttle, author of The World Peace Diet

You are what you eat, but do you know what you're eating?

I look at cancer as a gift of healthy learning, but some of the things I've learned are quite disturbing and disheartening. Sadly, there are a lot of things happening in our world today that could have devastating effects on how long we live and what conditions we live in. We are only uncovering the start of what the next generations will see and endure, unless we all make some serious changes to how we live.

I'm talking about the changes in our food supply due to the mass production and processed foods. I know this is a difficult topic and many people "don't want to know" as they feel it's too hard to change and nothing will help anyway. I believe it can and will change. **Together we are billions of people. We can make a difference by our choices.**

Money and power have become such huge directors in our society and our food supply. These are two of the biggest reasons our food supply is in the state it's in and getting worse. Food manufacturers are receiving large monetary benefits while providing unhealthy, processed foods and using creative advertising to entice purchases. Look at the word "natural". It's constantly used on packaging, but it doesn't necessarily provide good nutrition. There are no regulations or criteria required to use it. How many times have you been enticed to buy something because it says "natural"? I was and still am sometimes.

The difference now is that I have more knowledge and can read the ingredient label. For example, a product labelled "all natural" cannot contain added colour, artificial flavouring, or synthetic substances. However, these products can contain natural flavouring, colour, additives and preservatives, which are all produced in a lab. They can also contain various processed sweeteners. Our body has to work so hard to digest these products. Why eat these foods and challenge your system when eating food the way Mother Nature intended is what the body needs and thrives on?

Food is contributing to a very sick world. The reality is that our food supply doesn't provide the nutrients that it used to and this is a big factor in why people are getting sick. The pesticides and toxins used in conventional farming are leaving chemical residue in your food, soil and water.

The Environmental Protection Agency reports that the majority of pesticides now in use are *probable or possible cancer causers*. Studies of farm workers who work with pesticides suggest a link between pesticide use and brain cancer, Parkinson's disease and various other cancers.

Organic is the way Mother Nature intended food to be and is the only word that requires actual certification and documented standards. Organic farmers are required to follow strict farming processes that do not include the use of pesticides, genetically modified organisms, chemical fertilizers, hormones and antibiotics when raising livestock or growing crops. Most people see organic farming as the producer of healthy food, but protecting the environment and minimizing soil degradation is also a huge part of organic farming. They help preserve the land and water for future generations. We need healthy soil and clean water to grow healthy crops.

BENEFITS OF ORGANIC FOOD:

- Grown without Genetically Modified Organisms
- Animals are not fed antibiotics or growth hormone
- Healthy soil due to regular crop rotation = more vitamins and minerals
- Safer for farmers as long term exposure to high dose pesticides can increase health risk
- Local organic farming eliminates transportation from other countries reducing pollution
- Local organic will mean you will be eating "in season" fruits and vegetables, the way our ancestors used to eat. Just buy extra and freeze them so you will have them available all year

---

There will be several local organic farms in your area and some will offer farm tours so you can see the process and care that is taken in growing your food. I recently visited one north of Toronto and it inspired me to find out how I can grow my own food next summer. Standing in a field with rows and rows of healthy food all around me grown without the use of harmful chemicals gave me hope that our food supply can be healthy again. It's really important. Locally grown can also be very healthy. There are some local farmers who still farm their land the old fashioned way, similar to organic farms, but without certification. Talk to your local farmers, ask what their process is, and how they feel about mass food production. True farmers take pride in their land and the food they supply....they will probably be thrilled to show you around and help educate you.

Another reason to look for organic or locally grown is Irradiation. Did you know that some non-organic fruits and vegetables are irradiated to keep them from going bad during transportation? Irradiation exposes food to bursts of gamma rays, x-rays or electron beams. Common irradiated foods are onions, potatoes, wheat, flour, whole wheat, spices, and dehydrated seasonings. Although many government agencies have agreed this *appears* to be a safe practice, it has been noted that irradiation can result in loss of nutrients. Another concern is that irradiation can be used to cover up poor farming or sanitation practices and can also create small amounts of cancer causing compounds in each food.

Organic foods cannot be irradiated. While they debate whether using this process on the food is potentially dangerous to human health, I prefer to buy organic whenever possible and just know for sure that I'm eating the healthiest food available. Hopefully soon I will be able to grow my own.

I know it can be expensive to buy organic so simply refer to the *Dirty Dozen* and *Clean Fifteen* lists on the next page to ensure you are, at least, doing the best you can for you and your family. The "Dirty Dozen" are foods that have been found to have high amounts of pesticide residue and should be purchased organic if possible. "Clean Fifteen" are foods that can be bought conventionally.

This list is provided and updated regularly on the Environmental Working Group website. It's an awesome resource for many pesticides and chemicals contaminating our food and products. Check it out if you haven't already done so.

2014 Updated Lists

Dirty Dozen	**Clean Fifteen**
Apple	Avocados
Strawberries	Sweet corn (beware of GMO)
Grapes	Pineapple
Celery	Cabbage
Peaches	Sweet peas (frozen)
Spinach	Onions
Sweet bell peppers	Asparagus
Nectarines (imported)	Mangos
Cucumbers	Papayas
Cherry Tomatoes	Kiwi
Snap peas (imported)	Eggplant
Potatoes	Grapefruit
	Cantaloupe
Plus 2 extra:	Cauliflower
Hot peppers	Sweet potatoes
Kale/collard greens	

Another little tip to know when you're shopping to ensure you are getting the organic produce, check the PLU number. This is the 5-digit PLU number found on the sticker attached to the produce and will start with:

9 = ORGANIC (5 digit code, Eg. 94135 is on my Royal Gala apples)

3 = CONVENTIONALLY GROWN (4 digit code starting with 3)

4 = CONVENTIONALLY GROWN (4 digit code starting with 4)

It's always good to check the PLU sticker on the actual product. I picked up an apple from the organic section recently and got back to work only to find the PLU started with 4. I went back and exchanged it for a 9.

8 = GMO (Genetically Modified Organisms), not yet in use

This was setup for future use when GMO labelling is required

GENETICALLY MODIFIED ORGANISMS:

I had never heard the term genetically modified organisms or GMOs before my diagnosis. The spring after my surgery, I attended a conference in California called the Longevity Now Conference hosted by David Wolfe, world-renowned nutrition expert. Since I was back on my healthy path after the infection, this seemed like a great learning environment. It was at this conference that I first learned about GMOs.

I was shocked to hear that my food was being scientifically modified. During the conference I learned that GMOs are produced in a lab. That in itself concerned me. It's disturbing to think about the process of taking genes/DNA from a species and inserting into another in a petri dish.

In addition to what is being combined together in the lab, they also add another ingredient called Round-Up Ready. It's the herbicide farmers spray the crops with. Injecting it into the seed allows the crop to be resistant to the spray. I listened intently to the speakers at the conference as they shared valuable information. GMOs didn't sound healthy to me and it was something that I had been simply unaware of. Our "food" is being grown with herbicide in it. How could this be possible?

The same company that produces Round-up Ready herbicide also produces GMO seeds. They create the GMO seeds the farmers have to pay for each year, and also provide the Roundup Ready herbicide to spray and kill weeds. This same company hold patents on all of it.

In other industries this would be a conflict of interest and questionable safety. Independent lab studies have shown GMOs are linked to allergies, digestion issues, reproductive and fertility problems, compromised immune system (which we learned earlier is a precursor to disease), and autism to name a few. Although there is no scientific proof on these links *yet*, it's hard not to question the rise in these health issues along with the increase in GMO ingredients in our food.

GMO STATISTICS:

Approximately 80-90% of all packaged products in the grocery store contain GMO ingredients. Here is a list of the foods that are predominately GMO and you will find them in most packaged foods:

Soy = 94%

Cotton = 90%

Canola = 90%

Sugar Beets = 95% (FYI – 55% of sugar produced in US is genetically modified)

Corn = 88%

Hawaiian Papaya = 50%

WHAT CAN YOU DO?

- Do your own research. Being aware and understanding what is in our food is the first step.

- Read labels. Look for the ingredients that I've listed above. For example, most oils contain canola or corn so they would likely be GMO.

- Buy organic. Visit an Organic farm to see first-hand the care they take in growing your food.

You can imagine my surprise when I discovered that corn was 88% genetically modified. Popcorn was always my healthy snack prior to diagnosis. Now I know that bag of microwave popcorn was not only full of chemicals, but it also contained genetically modified corn. Sadly, I had no idea what I was giving my body.

We need to educate others and ourselves. I have been sharing information on GMOs in my seminars and always find people who, like me prior to the conference, are simply unaware that GMOs exist. The labelling of GMOs will be a great first step towards change, so we can make our own choice about the food we eat. Some manufacturers are proud to label their products as GMO free, allowing consumers to make that choice. This is extremely important to our future.

64 countries currently require GMO labelling or have implemented a complete ban. Unfortunately, Canada and United States have not yet followed suit. I am confident that we will see this change. Several US states have already made progress towards future labelling. Our power is in the money we spend and how we spend it.
Invest in your future. Make your health a priority. Avoid genetically modified foods.

Chapter 8

Juice and Smoothie Ideas for Detox and Healing

Juicing and blending is an easy way to give your body high doses of vitamins and minerals. I include a green powder drink containing chlorella, spirulina, or wheatgrass to assist my body with PH level or juice consisting of spinach, celery, parsley, cilantro, cucumber, lemon, ginger every day. This is to ensure I continue to thrive and keep my body at optimal health. I sometimes take my juicer with me to visit my family and it becomes a fun thing to do with my niece/nephew. Although they don't care for my green juice, I can usually get them to drink something with carrots or apples.

Each time we make juice together I know I'm sharing my gift of learning with them too. They will grow up with awareness of healthy nutrition, even if they are not keen on pure green juice yet. Educating our youth, now, will help them prevent disease in the future.

I've included some of my favourite juice/smoothie recipes I've found over the years. Some I've thrown together and some are based on amazing concoctions I've had at incredible juice bars or raw food restaurants around the world.

DIFFERENCE BETWEEN JUICING AND BLENDING

JUICING:
MY JACK LALANNE JUICER:

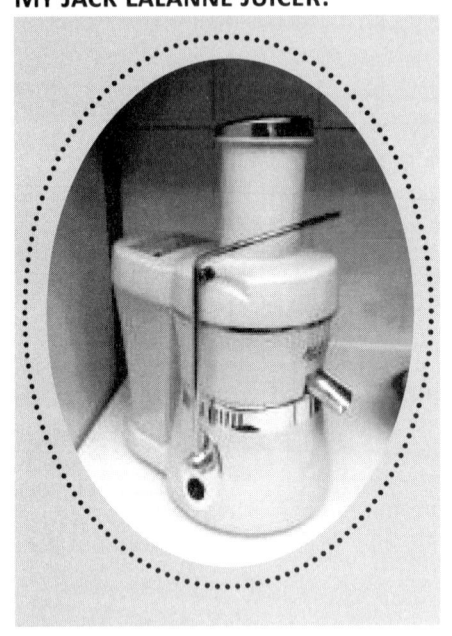

Juicing is the processing of vegetables and fruits through a juicer to remove pulp fibre. Only soluble (dissolves in water in your body) fibre remains, which allows the body to deliver easily absorbable nutrients into the bloodstream. This process limits the energy required in the digestion process. It takes a lot of vegetables to make 1 glass of juice so the nutrient values are huge.

Important Note: Be careful when juicing fruits, you will receive a high concentration of sugar and without the insoluble fibre to slow down the uptake you can experience a sugar spike.

HERE ARE SOME SUGAR VALUES TO CONSIDER:

1 Small apple = 10 grams of sugar
1 Small orange = 9 grams of sugar
1 Carrot = 5 grams of sugar
1 Beet = 7 grams of sugar

So if you've ever watched juice being made at a juice bar, they love to put in lots of apples, beets or carrots. Sometimes 2-4 each beverage, why? All these products deliver lots of juice/liquid, whereas, they have to use a lot of green vegetables to make up a glass and fruit adds flavour. That can add up to 20-30 grams of sugar in 1 glass of juice.

Compare that to 1- 8 oz. can of Pepsi, which is 27 grams of sugar. Now, don't get me wrong, these foods have nutritional values compared to a soft drink, but I tend to stick with my own juicer and mostly green vegetables so I can control the sugar.

Yes, my juice is always very green. Add some Cucumber and celery to your spinach/greens and you'll have lots of juice. If you do buy from a juice bar, ask them if they can accommodate you with more green vegetables.

BLENDING:
MY VITAMIX:

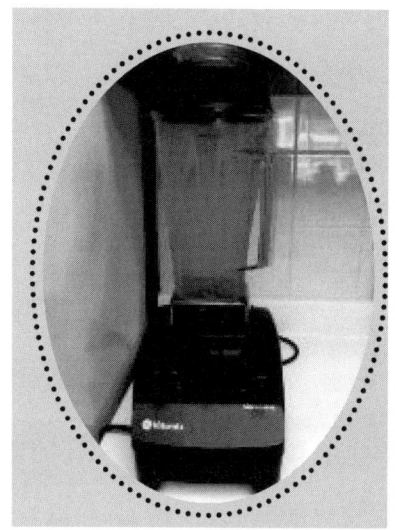

All ingredients are simply blended together in a high-speed blender. I love my Vitamix blender, but any high-speed blender is fine.

The smoothie retains both soluble and insoluble fibre. Insoluble fibre does not breakdown in water, but helps move food through the digestion process. This allows for a slower release of nutrients into the body. You won't absorb all the nutrients like juicing, but keeping the fibre is great for bowel health.

Added bonus to Blending: You can blend other options into the smoothie that you can't add to juice like protein powder, good fats like avocado or coconut, or awesome cancer fighting foods like burdock root or turmeric root. These are both in my morning smoothie.

Another great option if you have a high-speed blender like a Vitamix, is you can make a warm soup from pure vegetables. This is great for those days when you don't have time to prepare a homemade soup.

Before we get to my favourite juice recipes, let's look at some of the most common vegetables that are regularly used in healthy juice, smoothie, broth/soup and full meal recipes. I've compiled a list of amazing vegetables and teas from all my learning and tasting that I use regularly and the body system they can assist for overall health and wellness.

I've also included the emotion attached to each organ according to the Chinese Medicine chart we discussed earlier in the book

The gift of cancer helped me understand that emotions are a healthy part of life. During times of emotional stress, the body needs support, not fast food, sugar, or alcohol. These choices are often an emotional reaction and only make the body work even harder during a challenging time. In times like these your body really needs great nutrition.

Since my diagnosis, I am fascinated by Chinese Medicine and its doctrine that healing power is determined by our choices. I look forward to learning more ways to recognize the signs of emotional stress before physical signs are present.

Body awareness and prevention techniques are key. Take every opportunity to support your body and it will reward you with long-term optimal health.

Here's a quick reference guide so you can create your own fabulous healthy drinks, blended soups and full meals to help maintain optimal health for your body.

LIVER SUPPORT

Liver Support: Fruits, Vegetables, Herbs, Other	Apple, Asparagus, Avocado, Beet, Berries, Broccoli, Burdock Root, Cabbage, Carrot, Cauliflower, Celery, Dandelion Root/Leaf, Garlic, Grapefruit, Kale, Lemon, Onion, Seaweed (Wakame, Dulse, Nori), Spinach, Tomato, Turmeric Root, Walnuts, Milk Thistle tincture, Turmeric tincture Tinctures are liquid herbal extracts easily added to a glass of water. I use St. Francis as they are recognized worldwide for their high standards and excellent products.
Liver Support: Teas	Green Tea/Matcha Tea, Dandelion Tea, Burdock Root Tea, Milk Thistle Tea

Chinese medicine emotional link

Anger and frustration can affect the liver so at these times I ensure I incorporate a variety of these foods to support my liver.

KIDNEY SUPPORT

Kidney Support: Fruits, Vegetables, Herbs, Other	Apple, Asparagus, Avocado, Beets, Berries, Broccoli, Burdock Root, Cabbage, Carrot, Cauliflower, Celery, Cranberries, Cucumber, Fennel Root, Garlic, Ginger, Grapes, Green Beans, Kidney Beans, Lemon, Onion, Parsley, Red Bell Pepper, Seaweed (Wakame, Dulse, Nori), Spinach, Turmeric Root, Watermelon
Kidney Support: Teas	Water *Sufficient water is crucial to good Kidney function Green Tea/Matcha Tea, Dandelion Tea, Stinging Nettle, Marshmallow Root Tea

Chinese medicine emotional link

Fear is connected to the kidneys so these foods along with calming meditation will help bring kidneys back into balance.

HEART SUPPORT

Heart Support: Fruits, Vegetables, Herbs, Other	Apple, Asparagus, Beets, Berries, Carrot, Cayenne, Celery, Dandelion Root, Garlic, Ginger, Green Leafy (Kale, Spinach), Lemon, Onion, Pomegranate, Radish, Red Grapes, Squash, Tomatoes, Turmeric Root
Heart Support: Teas	Green Tea/Matcha Tea, Rooibos Tea, Hawthorn Berry, Hibiscus Tea

Chinese medicine emotional link:

The heart is attached to joy. We all need a healthy dose of joy in our life on a regular basis. Without it, the body isn't working as a whole unit. Including these foods will help keep the heart strong for those, hopefully few times, when joy is missing in your life.

LUNG SUPPORT

Lung Support: Fruits, Vegetables, Herbs, Other	Apple, Beans (Kidney, Pinto, Black), Berries, Bok Choy, Broccoli, Cabbage, Carrot, Cayenne, Cauliflower, Cinnamon, Garlic, Ginger, Grapefruit, Kale, Kiwi, Lemon Water, Lentils, Onion, Orange, Oregano, Pomegranate, Radish, Sage, Thyme, Turmeric, Walnuts
Lung Support: Teas	Green Tea/Matcha Tea, Black Tea, Licorice Root, Peppermint

Chinese medicine emotional link

Grief/Sadness are emotions that come with a variety of different losses that are a part of life. During these times, opt for some of these food options and some deep breathing exercises to nourish the lungs

SPLEEN & STOMACH SUPPORT

Spleen and Stomach Support: Fruits, Vegetables, Herbs, Other *Note:* The Spleen likes mainly cooked/warmed foods so a great way to get your "juice" is to boil a bunch of vegetables for a couple minutes then let simmer covered for 10 min and drink the broth.	Beets, Berries, Broccoli, Cabbage, Carrot, Celery, Cinnamon, Cucumbers, Dandelion Root/Leaf, Eggplant, Fennel, Garlic, Green Leafy (Kale, Spinach), Ginger, Lemon Water, Maitake/Shitake Mushrooms, Onion, Orange, Nutmeg, Pumpkin, Radish, Squash, Sweet Potatoes
Spleen and Stomach Support: Teas	Dandelion Tea, Sorrel Tea, Ginger Tea, Fennel Tea

Chinese medicine emotional link:

Anxiety and worry affect most of us probably more regularly than we realize. This can potentially affect the Spleen and compromise our immune system. We need to offer the body some assistance. These foods combined with Tai Chi or meditation definitely help.

SKIN NUTRIENTS

Skin Nutrient/Support: Fruits, Vegetables, Herbs, Other	Acai, Almonds, Avocado, Beets, Berries, Brazil Nuts, Broccoli, Burdock Root, Carrots, Coconuts/Oil, Cucumber, Dandelion Root/Leaf, Garlic, Kale, Kiwi, Parsley, Pineapple, Pumpkin, Spinach, Sunflower Seeds, Sweet Potatoes, Tomatoes, Turmeric, Walnuts, Water
Skin Nutrient/Support: Teas	Green Tea/Matcha Tea, Seabuckthorn Tea
Your skin reflects your inner health	

Juice and Smoothie Recipes

My Morning Power Boost Smoothie

Tools
Blender

Ingredients
1 handful of spinach
1 celery stock
2 inch burdock root peeled
½ inch turmeric root
1 tsp. sea vegetables or Vitamineral Greens
½ tsp. spirulina
Sunwarrior vegan protein (Optional)
¼-½ cup water or ice for liquid consistency

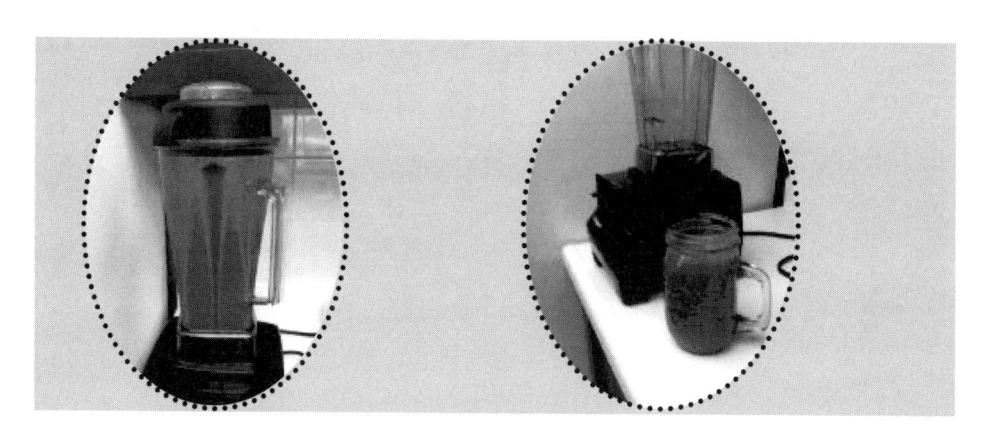

Vitamix in action!

Nutrient filled green smoothie

Preparation (blender)
Combine ingredients into blender.
Blend on high until liquid consistency is apparent and pour into glass.

Be Well Smoothie or Juice

Tools
Blender or Juicer

Ingredients
1 handful of spinach
1 handful of kale
½ cucumber
Small piece of fresh ginger (to taste)
1 lemon (squeezed for juice)
¼-½ cup water or ice (smoothie preparation)

Preparation (blender)
Combine ingredients into blender.
Blend on high until liquid consistency is apparent and pour into glass.

Preparation (juicer)
Juice each item through juicer and pour into glass and serve.

Clear Skin Smoothie or Juice

Tools

Blender or Juicer

Ingredients

1 handful kale
1 handful spinach
½ cucumber
1 handful parsley
¼-½ cup water or ice (smoothie preparation)

Preparation (blender)
Combine ingredients into blender.
Blend on high until liquid consistency is apparent and pour into glass.

Preparation (juicer)
Juice each item through juicer and pour into glass and serve.

Beet The Day Smoothie or Juice

Tools
Blender or Juicer

Ingredientsa
1 handful spinach
½ cucumber
1 celery stock
1 beet
½ cup blueberries
1 scoop protein powder (optional with smoothie)
¼-½ cup water or ice (smoothie preparation)

Preparation (blender)
Combine ingredients into blender.
Blend on high until liquid consistency is apparent and pour into glass.

Preparation (juicer)
Juice each item through juicer and pour into glass and serve.

Optimal Cleanse

Tools
Blender or Juicer

Ingredients
1 handful spinach
1 cucumber
1 celery stock
½ inch turmeric root
½ handful mint leaves
1 lemon (squeezed for juice)
¼-½ cup water (smoothie preparation)

Preparation (blender)
Combine ingredients into blender.
Blend on high until liquid consistency is apparent and pour into glass.

Preparation (juicer)
Juice each item through juicer and pour into glass and serve.

Happy Liver Juice

Tools
Blender or Juicer

Ingredients
1 handful spinach
½-1 small handful dandelion leaf (note: this is bitter so go easy at first)
½ inch burdock root
1 carrot
1 celery stock
½ inch turmeric root
1 apple (if needed for sweetness…but remember the sugar content in fruits/carrots can add up!)
¼-½ cup water or ice (smoothie preparation)

Preparation (blender)
Combine ingredients into blender.
Blend on high until liquid consistency is apparent and pour into glass.

Preparation (juicer)
Juice each item through juicer and pour into glass and serve.

Kidney Assistant Juice

Tools
Blender or Juicer

Ingredients
3 cups purple cabbage or regular cabbage
1 fennel head
1 celery stock
1 handful of parsley
½ cucumber
¼-½ cup water or ice (smoothie preparation)

Preparation (blender)
Combine ingredients into blender.
Blend on high until liquid consistency is apparent and pour into glass.

Preparation (juicer)
Juice each item through juicer and pour into glass and serve.

Heart Be Strong

Tools
Blender or Juicer

Ingredients
1 beet
1 handful kale or spinach
1 celery stock
½ inch turmeric root
1 small handful of dandelion leaf (This is bitter so go easy on the amount)
¼ inch ginger root (to taste as this can be overpowering)
¼-½ cup water or ice (smoothie preparation)

Preparation (blender)
Combine ingredients into blender.
Blend on high until liquid consistency is apparent and pour into glass.

Preparation (juicer)
Juice each item through juicer and pour into glass and serve.

Lungs Are For Living

Tools
Blender or Juicer

Ingredients
1 handful kale
1 carrot
1 celery stock
½ inch ginger (to taste)
1 handful cabbage
2 radish
¼-½ cup water or ice (smoothie preparation)

Preparation (blender)
Combine ingredients into blender.
Blend on high until liquid consistency is apparent and pour into glass.

Preparation (juicer)
Juice each item through juicer and pour into glass and serve.

Wheatgrass

Wheatgrass is another great addition to any juice or smoothie. If you don't have an actual wheatgrass juicer you can buy wheatgrass that has been "flash-frozen" in cubes. Most high-end health food stores will carry them or there are also powdered wheatgrass options.

Wheatgrass is high in Chlorophyll that cleanses and builds the blood. Chlorophyll has high levels of oxygen along with numerous nutrients. Oxygenated cells is a huge factor in disease prevention and keeping the body healthy (See exercise chapter for more information).

Cheers to your morning wheatgrass shot!

Spirulina

Spirulina is one of the best superfoods out there. It's not the tastiest, but if you can get past the taste, this Algae is amazing. High in protein, essential fatty acids, vitamins, and minerals, as it's known as a "complete" food. Adding this to your morning smoothie or stir it into your juice will have an incredible impact on your overall health.

As noted, the recipes I've included above can be either juiced or prepared as a smoothie in a high-speed blender like a Vitamix. These recipes are just guidelines based on trial and error. Trust me sometimes those trials, left little to be desired! Use whatever appliance you have available and alter the recipe accordingly. You probably noticed I haven't used a lot of fruits in the recipes. I'm always very aware of the sugar content when preparing any foods. Although fruits are good for you, we still need to remember sugar has a huge role in many diseases, so everything in moderation. Yes, even in fresh juices.

Have fun making your own fabulous juice/smoothie concoctions!

Chapter 9

Recipe Ideas for Optimal Health

Raw food is known to have a high nutrient content as it contains live enzymes that help digest food. Cooking food at high temperatures can destroy live enzymes resulting in reduced nutrients for the body to absorb. Food is still considered raw and will retain enzymes and nutrients if kept under 115°F. This can be done with a dehydrator, a must have kitchen tool for anyone who likes snacks.

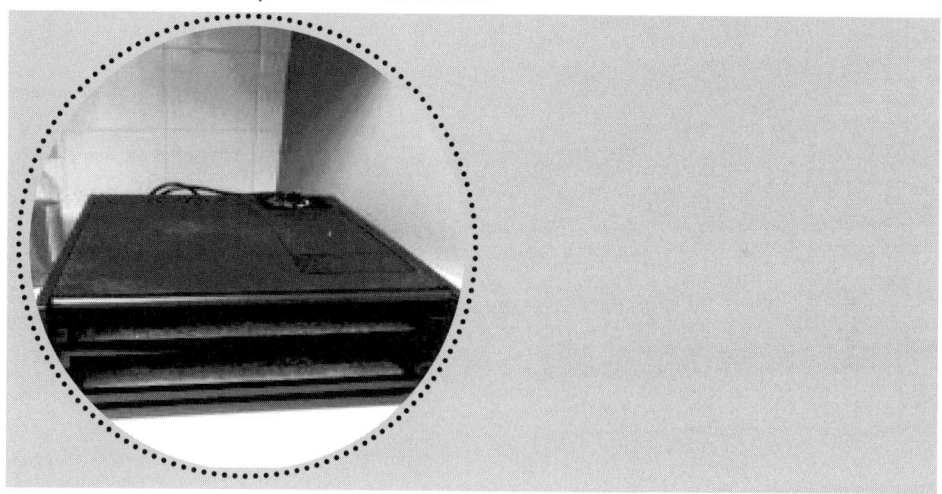

You can make crackers, bread, chips, and dried vegetables/fruits. Dehydrated foods gives a great option to the processed products available in grocery stores. Your family will love them!

Another great tool for raw food preparation is a Spiralizer. This will allow you to make pasta from zucchini and other vegetables. The picture below shows zucchini and squash.

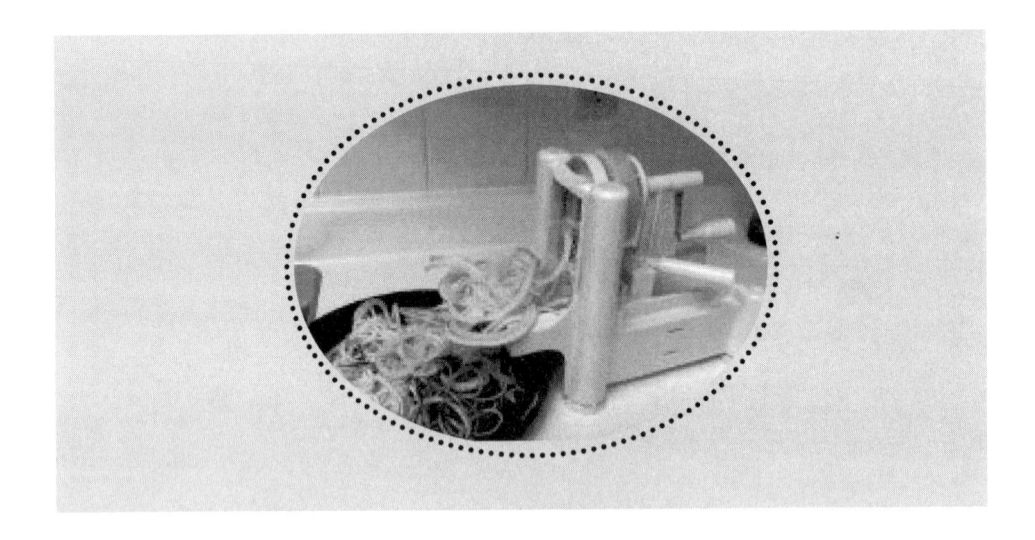

I've included some of my absolute favourite raw food recipes below. I maintain eating about 70% raw food and the rest is cooked. I make some amazing soups in my Vitamix, dehydrate flax crackers, kale and zucchini chips that are all still considered raw food. As you can see my gift of learning has brought me some incredible information. I never used any spices and now I've learned that any food can taste amazing just by the spices you use. Oregano, garlic, onion, cayenne…..all flavours that are amazing on these foods!

RAW BREAKFAST OPTIONS

Selene's Protein Source (from my cancer protocol)

Tools
Nut grinder
4 – 6 small glass (freezer safe) containers

Ingredients
¼ cup almonds
¼ cup cashews
¼ cup brazil nuts
¼ cup sunflower seeds
¼ cup flax seeds
2 tbsp. organic apple juice

Preparation
Combine almonds, cashews, brazil nuts, sunflower seeds and flax seeds into nut grinder and grind to powder.

In small glass containers add 2 tbsp. of the powdered nut mixture to each container (should make approximately 4-6 containers).

Add organic apple juice to each one and stir.

Cover containers and place in freezer to ferment.

Each morning simply add hot water and you have a great protein source in a yummy cereal.

Almost "Scrambled" Eggs

Tools
Blender

Ingredients
1 cup almonds/brazil nuts/walnuts (equal parts)
½ cup sunflower seeds
1 tsp. turmeric
½ cup water
1 handful parsley
1 handful cilantro
½ cup chopped tomato
1 chopped small green onion
¼ tsp. sea salt to taste

Pre-Prep
Soak almonds, brazil nuts, walnuts and sunflower seeds in water (at room temperature) for 2 hours before beginning. Rinsing a few times within the 2 hours. Soaking makes the nuts more easily digestible by the body and therefore more nutrients can be absorbed.

Preparation
Combine nuts, seeds, salt, and turmeric, into blender and chop until mixed.

Add parsley, cilantro, tomato, onion to mixture and blend/chop on medium to scrambled egg consistency.

Serve just like scrambled eggs!

Homemade Granola

Tools
Nut Grinder

Ingredients
½ cup walnuts
½ cup almonds
½ cup sunflower seeds
½ cup pumpkin seeds
½ cup flax seeds (process lightly to chop but not to powder)
1 tbsp. raisins
¼ cup blueberries
1 tbsp. hemp hearts
1 tsp. raw coconut
1 pinch of cinnamon and nutmeg to taste
1 cup hot water

Optional
1 handful of chia seeds

Preparation
Combine walnuts, almonds, sunflower seeds, pumpkin seeds and flax seeds into nut grinder and lightly chop but not to powder.

Add 1 cup of hot water.

If you want to make this more like porridge, just add handful of chia seeds and they will expand to a gel like texture and combine the ingredients together.

Holy Crap!

Don't have time to prepare breakfast? There is a healthy store bought option from a company called Holy Crap. All organic ingredients, nothing but real food.

Ingredients
chia
buckwheat
hemp seeds
raisins
dried cranberries
apple bits
cinnamon

Preparation
Simply add 1 cup of water (I like warm water) or liquid of your choice, let soak for 5 min to allow chia seeds to become a gel-like consistency.
They also have a version called Skinny B that is chia, buckwheat, and hemp seeds. Add in a few blueberries and it's a fabulous quick breakfast.

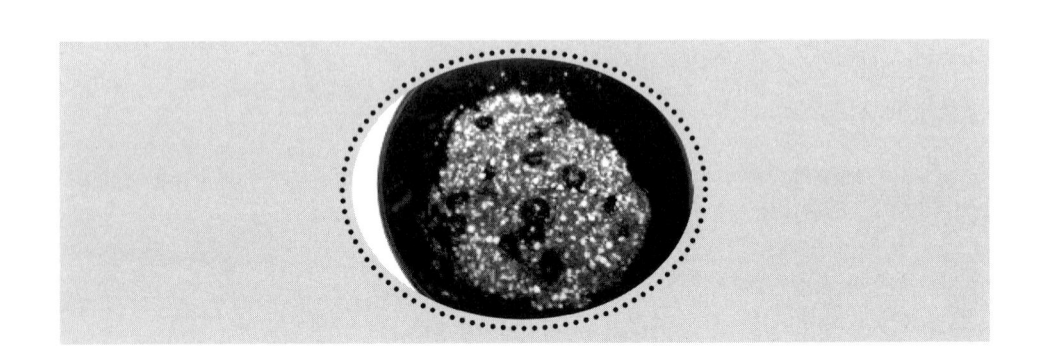

Raw Lunch and Dinner Options

Cleansing Green Soup

Tools
Blender

Ingredients
½-1 avocado
1 cup kale or spinach
1 cucumbers
1 lemon (squeezed for juice)
1 pinch of ginger to taste…go easy…not everyone loves this powerful taste
1 celery stalk
1 clove garlic (to taste preference)
1 green onion
½ tsp. of sea salt

Preparation
Combine ingredients into blender.
Blend on high until soup consistency is apparent. Pour into bowl and enjoy.

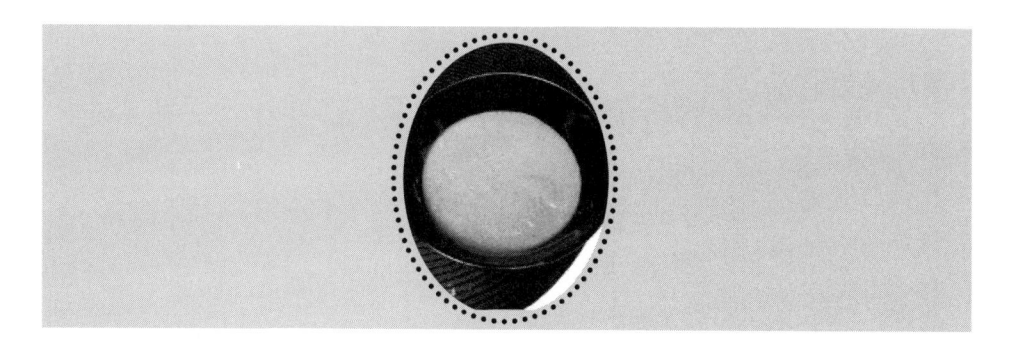

Raw Carrot Soup

Tools
Blender

Ingredients
2 carrots chopped
½ cup soaked cashews (or nut of your choice, but cashews work really well)
1 tsp. oregano
½ cup water

1 pinch of sea salt to taste

Pre-Prep
Soak cashews (or nut of your choice) in water (at room temperature) for 2 hours before beginning. Rinse.

Preparation
Combine ingredients into blender.

Blend on high until soup consistency is apparent. Pour into bowl and enjoy!

Broccoli Soup

Tools
Blender

Ingredients
1 cup broccoli
½ cup soaked cashews
½ cup water
½ lemon (squeezed for juice)

Pre-Prep

Soak cashews in water (at room temperature) for 2 hours before beginning. Rinse.

Preparation

Combine ingredients into blender.

Blend on high until soup consistency is apparent. Pour into bowl and enjoy!

Want cheese on the broccoli soup? Here's a great little trick for raw Parmesan.

Raw Parmesan "Cheese"

Tools
Blender

Ingredients
½ cup raw cashews
½ cup nutritional yeast (deactivated yeast with a cheesy nutty flavor used in many vegan recipes, also a great source of B12)

Preparation
Combine ingredients into blender.

Blend on high until texture is like parmesan.

Keep in fridge for quick sprinkle on soups or Zucchini Pasta

Tomato/Garlic Soup

Tools
Blender

Ingredients
1 tomato
1 clove garlic
¼ cup soaked cashews
1 celery Stock
1 tsp. oregano
½ cup water

Pre-Prep
Soak cashews in water (at room temperature) for 2 hours before beginning. Rinse.

Preparation
Combine ingredients into blender.

Blend on high until soup consistency is apparent. Pour into bowl and enjoy.

"Raw" Garlic Mashed Potato

Tools
Blender

Ingredients
1 cauliflower head, chopped
1 lemon (squeezed for juice)
1 avocado
1 clove garlic
1 green onion, chopped
½ tsp. sea Salt

Optional
¼ cup nutritional yeast (adds flavour and nutrients)

Preparation
Combine ingredients into blender.

Blend on high until smooth and creamy consistency is apparent. Serve and enjoy!

Basil/Sun Dried "Cheese"

Tools
Blender

Ingredients
½ cup of sun dried tomatoes
3 cups cashews
2-3 lemons squeezed juice
1 handful basil leaves
½ green onion
1 clove garlic
½ tsp. sea salt

Optional

¼ cup nutritional yeast (adds flavour and nutrients)

Pre-Prep
Soak cashews and sun-dried tomatoes in water (at room temperature) for 1 hour before beginning. Rinse.

Preparation
Combine ingredients into blender.

Blend on high until smooth and creamy consistency is apparent.

Refrigerate and serve with yummy dehydrated flax crackers. Recipe below.

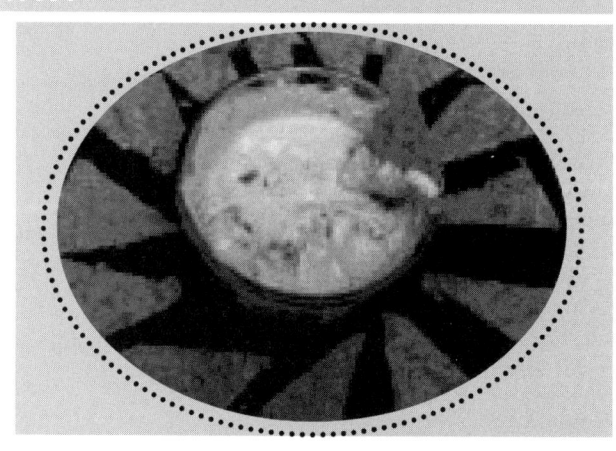

Dehydrated Flax Crackers

Tools
Dehydrator
Paraflax paper

Ingredients
1 cup of golden/brown flax seeds
½ cup sunflower and pumpkin seeds (equal parts)
1 chopped green onion
1 clove garlic
1 tsp. oregano
¼ tsp. sea salt
¾ cup of water

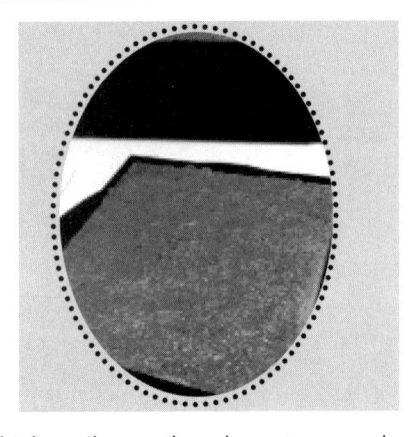

Preparation
Combine all ingredients into blender and blend on high until smooth and easy to spread.
Spread on paraflax sheets.
Turn dehydrator to 115°F and place sheets inside.
Dehydrate for 1 hour.
Remove from dehydrator and use knife to score the crackers to desired size.
Turn down dehydrator to 100°F/105°F and place sheets back inside to dehydrate for 6-8 hours.
Remove from dehydrator and let cool for 3-4 hours before removing parflax paper.
Turn crackers over and continue dehydrating until crackers are firm and crisp.

Butternut Pasta (or Zucchini Noodles)

Tools
Spiralizer cheese grater if Spiralizer not available

Ingredients
½ butternut squash or 1 full zucchini

Preparation
Spiral into noodles. If you don't have a turning slicer like I've shown below, simply grate the vegetable into noodles with cheese grater.

Tomato Sauce

Tools
Blender

Ingredients
3 tomatoes
½ cup sundried tomatoes
½ avocado
½ handful fresh basil leaves
2 cloves garlic
2 tbsp. olive oil
½ tsp. oregano
½ tsp. sea salt

Preparation

Combine ingredients into blender.

Blend on high until smooth and creamy consistency is apparent. Serve and enjoy!

Buying a Spiralizer was a great investment. In a couple of minutes I made squash and zucchini noodles.

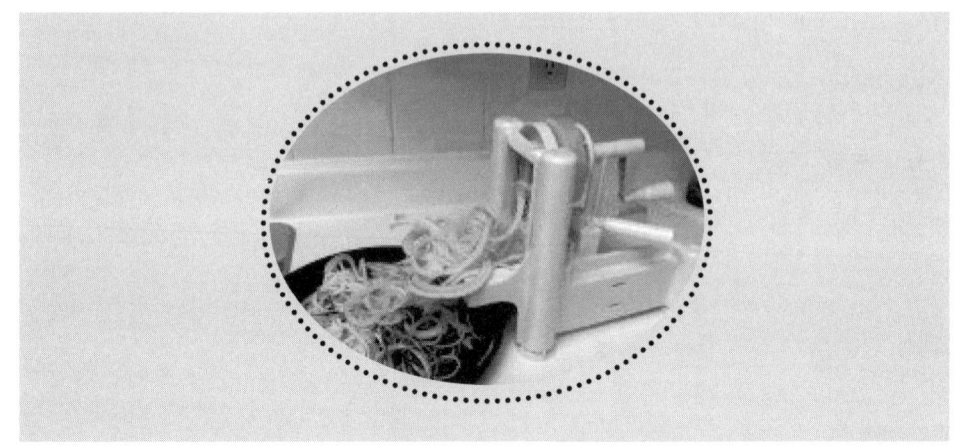

Delicious plate of Zucchini, Squash, and Kelp noodles with sunflower sprouts, broccoli and a yummy sauce, takes just 5 minutes!

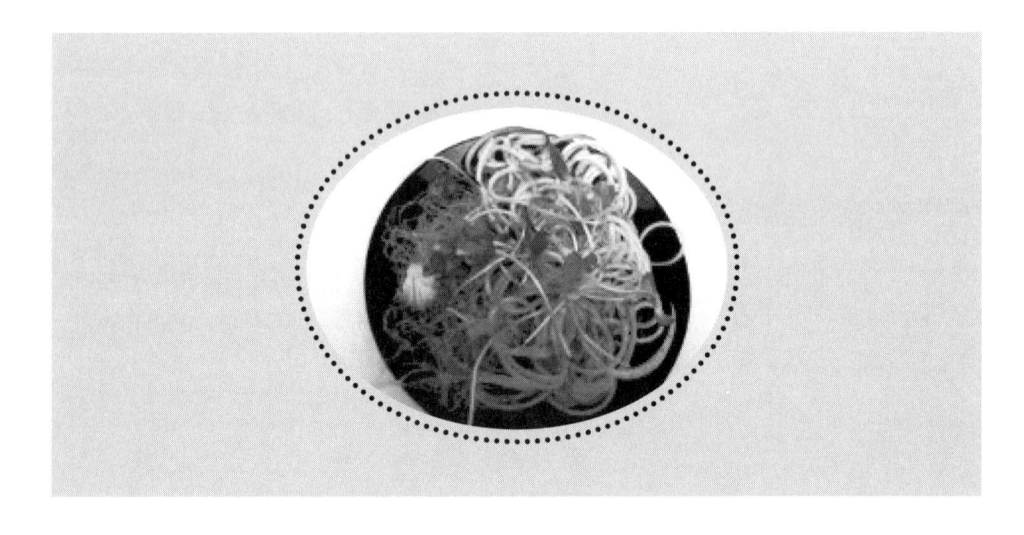

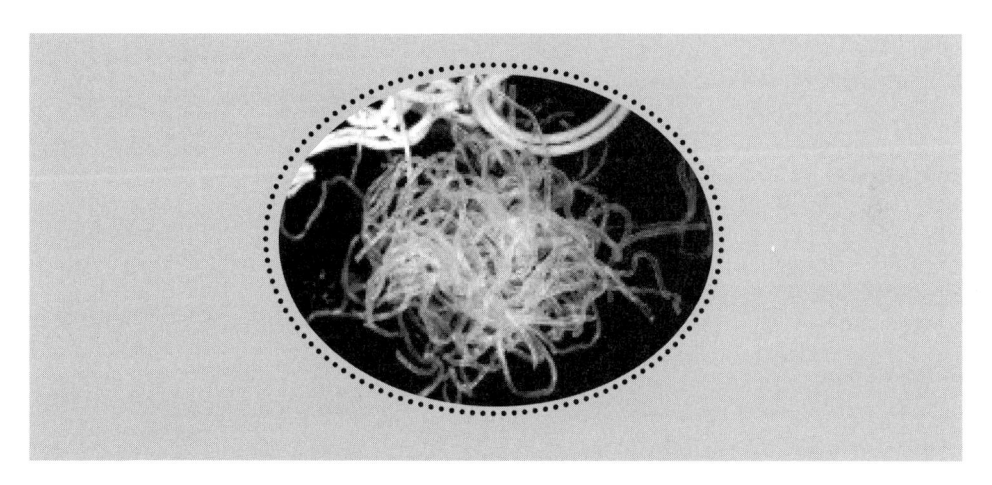

KELP NOODLES

Kelp noodles are very versatile. With over 70 nutrients and minerals, this little Algae powerhouse is a great addition to any salad or pasta (as in the pasta shown above). It has a rather bland taste so you can flavour with any sauce or spice. Packaged in water and available in healthy food stores. Regular grocery stores don't usually carry them.

Walnut "Meatballs"

Tools
Blender

Ingredients
1 cup walnuts
1 tbsp. nutritional yeast
1 tbsp. olive oil
2 tsp. fresh lemon juice
2 tsp. Nama Shoyu soy sauce
1 tsp. garlic minced or dried
1 tsp. green onion
1 ½ tsp. parsley

Pre-Prep
Soak walnuts in water (at room temperature) for 2 hour before beginning. Rinse.

Preparation
Combine ingredients into blender.

Blend alternating medium and high until smooth consistency is apparent.

Use a spoon to scoop mixture and form small "meatballs".

Serve and enjoy!

Spinach and "Cheese" Portobello Mushrooms

Tools
Blender

Ingredients
6 large portobello mushrooms
2 tbsp. olive oil
1 tsp. oregano
1 clove garlic
1 green onion
1 pinch of sea salt to taste
1 tbsp. fresh lemon juice

Preparation
Combine all ingredients except mushrooms into bowl and mix well. Set mushrooms in bowl with mixture and let sit for 30-60 minutes.

Prepare Spinach/Cheese

Tools
Blender
Dehydrator

Ingredients
1 cup soaked cashews/walnuts (equal parts)
1 clove garlic
1 green onion
2 cups spinach
1 handful basil
1 lemon (squeezed for juice)

Pre-Prep
Soak walnuts and cashews in water (at room temperature) for 2 hour before beginning. Rinse.

Preparation
Combine all ingredients in blender.

Blend on high until smooth and creamy consistency is apparent.

Fill each Portobello mushroom evenly with cheese

Place in dehydrator and dehydrate for 3 hours on 115 F. I've only done this in a dehydrator, but I'm sure you could put these in the oven on low for less time. Serve and enjoy!

Nori Rolls

Ingredients
8 nori sheets
2 cups spinach
1 cucumber
1 celery stalk
1 carrot
1 handful sunflower sprouts
1 avocado

Preparation
Slice vegetables in small slices to place in the Nori sheets.

Lightly moisten sheets with water

Place and arrange veggies onto sheet and roll tightly.

Cut sheets at desired sizes to create a "sushi like" roll.

Orange, Ginger, Garlic dipping sauce

Tools
Blender

Ingredients
1 orange
1 clove garlic
½ inch ginger
¼ cup olive oil

Preparation
Combine ingredients into blender.
Blend on high until smooth consistency is apparent.

Serve with Nori Rolls for a fabulous dip.

Dehydrated Veggie Burger

Tools
Blender
Dehydrator
Paraflax paper

Ingredients
¼ cup walnuts
1/8 cup flax seeds
¼ cup sunflower seeds
¼ cup pumpkin seeds
1 clove garlic
1 green onion
½ lemon (squeezed for juice)
¼ cup hemp hearts
2 tbsp. chia seeds
¼ cup chopped celery
¼ cup chopped carrots
1 handful chopped parsley

Pre-Prep
Soak walnuts, sunflower seeds, flax seeds and pumpkin seeds in water (at room temperature) for 1 hour before beginning. Rinse.

Preparation
Combine walnuts, flax seeds, sunflower seeds, pumpkin seeds, garlic, onion and lemon juice in blender.

Blend alternating medium and high until smooth consistency is apparent.

Add hemp hearts, chia seeds, celery, carrots and parsley into blender.

Blend on high until all ingredients have been evenly broken up.

Use a spoon or your hands to form "veggie burgers" (should be flat and about ½" thick)

Turn dehydrator on to 115°F and place "veggie burgers" on paraflax sheets in the dehydrator for 1.5 hours.

Reduce temperature to 105°F and continue for approximately 5 hours.

Check half way through and if they are staying together remove paraflax paper and turn over.

Remove from dehydrator and serve.

Dehydrated "Bread-ish" Snacks

Tools
Nut grinder
Blender
Parchment paper

Ingredients
2 cups almonds/walnuts (equal parts)
1 cup flax seeds
1 ½ tbsp. olive oil
1 tbsp. dried basil
1 tbsp. oregano
1 pinch of sea salt to taste

Preparation
Combine almonds, walnuts and flax seeds into nut grinder and grind to powder.

Combine nut powder and olive oil, basil, oregano and sea salt into blender and blend on high until smooth consistency is apparent.

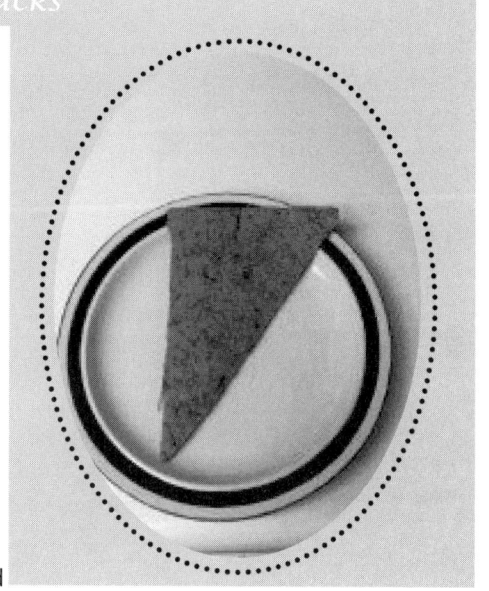

Spread on to parchment paper and dehydrate on 115°F for 1-2 hours.

Remove from dehydrator and score into desired shape and size.

Reduce temperature to 105°F and place back in dehydrator and continue dehydrating for 7-10 hours.

Halfway through dehydrating, remove parchment paper and turn over snacks.

Remove from dehydrator, serve and enjoy!

Dessert
We can't forget about dessert!

Choco-Ban Surprise

A really simple raw dessert that everybody loves is ice cream! Banana chocolate is a fan favourite.

Tools
Blender

Ingredients
2 frozen bananas
1 tsp. cacao or chocolate protein powder

Preparation
Combine ingredients into blender

Blend on high until creamy consistency is apparent.

Tastes just like ice cream! With frozen banana as the base you can create many different flavours using nuts, berries, vanilla, etc.

That's it for the "Raw Food" section. I hope you enjoy some of these recipes. They are so easy and so high in nutrients.

Cooked Food Recipes

This section is full of awesome cooked recipes to help keep the body warm, especially during winter months. These recipes are healthy, easy and quick to prepare. No need to stop and pick up a dinner with limited nutrition and toxins, when you can have a nutritious meal right at home.

Cooked Breakfast

Oatmeal Power

Tools
Small pot

Ingredients
½ cup steel cut oatmeal
1 handful berries
1 tbsp. sunflower seeds/pumpkin seeds (equal parts)
1 pinch of cinnamon

Preparation
Fill small pot with 2 cups of water and cook on high until boiling.

Add the oatmeal and stir.

Bring water back to a rolling boil before reducing heat to low.

Let oats simmer for 20-30 minutes, stirring occasionally.

When oats are tender and creamy remove from heat and add berries, sunflower seeds/pumpkin seeds and cinnamon.

It's a perfect way to start your day!

Morning Quinoa

Tools
Small pot

Ingredients
½ cup quinoa
½ banana
1 tbsp. almond butter
6-8 almonds/walnuts
1 handful blueberries
1 pinch of cinnamon (or any spice you prefer)

Preparation
Fill small pot with 1 ½ cups of water and cook on high until boiling.

Add the quinoa and stir.

Reduce temperature to med/low.

Cover and cook for about 12-15 minutes or until liquid is absorbed.

Remove from heat and let stand for 5 minutes.

Cut banana into small portions and add to quinoa.

Add almond butter, nuts blueberry and cinnamon.

Healthy Hearty Oatmeal

Oatmeal is a healthy option but why not jazz it up a little with some granola. Don't be deceived as granola sounds healthy, but the store bought brands are often quite high in fat, sugar and super calorific. Avoid the unnecessary calories and fat in many packaged versions by baking your own granola and/or muesli. It can be enjoyed on its own, as a snack or mix it with milk or yogurt with fresh fruit for breakfast. Thanks to my friend Jill Buckley and her sister for sharing this recipe. You can make it in advance and have it ready to go through the week.

Tools
Large bowl
Large baking sheet
Parchment paper

Ingredients
6 cups of rolled oats (the old-fashioned kind, not quick oats)
2 cups of chopped dried apricots, dates and/or prunes. - Raisins are tasty as well but add them in at the end or they will burn.
¾ cup honey or maple syrup (warm the honey slightly to make it easier to mix in)
1 tsp. each vanilla and cinnamon
¼ tsp. salt
½ cup sliced almonds
1/3 cup unsalted pumpkin seeds

Preparation
In the large bowl, mix all ingredients together

Line the large baking sheet with parchment paper and spread the mixture on it

Heat oven to 275°F and bake in the centre for about 1 hour, stirring twice, until light golden

Let the granola cool and it will become crunchy.

There are many great options to create your own amazing breakfast using the base of Oatmeal or Quinoa. Add a little pumpkin, cinnamon, ginger and nutmeg to have a pumpkin pie surprise! Or add a little apple and cinnamon to bring back the scent of apple pie. Spices can make a huge difference in the taste and they are so good for you.

How about a breakfast bar, prepared in advance, just waiting for you in the am? Breakfast is an important way to start your day, so if time is a factor try this tasty bar.

Breakfast Bar To Go!

Tools
Large bowl
Blender
Large baking sheet

Ingredients
2 cups oats
2 bananas
½ cup each of walnuts, almonds, sunflower and pumpkin seeds
2 tbsp hemp seeds
½ tsp. ginger
½ tsp. nutmeg

Preparation
In blender, process oats and nuts to a chopped consistency

Mix oats and nuts with all ingredients in large bowl until blended smoothly

Spread mixture on baking sheet and smooth out evenly covering the sheet.

Heat oven to 350°F and bake for 20-25 minutes.

Cool for 15 minutes, cut into bars and freeze. Voila, you have a perfect on the go breakfast.

Cooked Lunch and Dinner Options

Your body requires a combination of raw foods and cooked foods. Below are some healthy options to keep you warm and provide good nutrition. My good friend Jill Buckley, foodie extraordinaire, has shared some of her wonderful recipes below. She definitely has a knack for putting together some fantastic meals that are exceptionally healthy and balanced.

Selene's Daily Soup Recommendation (from my Cancer Protocol)

Tools
Large pot

Ingredients
4 cups water
6-12 garlic cloves
1 handful wakame seaweed
5-10 shiitake mushrooms (fresh or dry)
1 cup well-cooked grains or beans (I use quinoa or a combination of beans)
1 onion chopped up or you can put the whole thing in the pot
1 cup leeks chopped up
1-2 burdock roots (also called gobo)
1 turmeric root

Optional

1/3 cup miso

Preparation

Heat water on high until boiling and add all ingredients

Reduce heat to med/low, cover and let simmer

Add Miso if desired after other vegetables have cooked in the water.

Butternut Squash Soup

Soup it up! I always love a hot bowl of soup on a cold day. Soup is simple to prepare and can be made in large volumes that are easily stored or frozen.

Tools
Large pan

Ingredients
900g (2lb) fresh butternut squash
3 celery sticks, sliced
2 medium onion, chopped
1 garlic clove, crushed
2 tsp. chopped fresh lemon thyme
1 litre vegetable stock
2 bay Leaves
salt and freshly ground black pepper to taste
2 tbsp fat-free fromage frais (you could also use fat free sour cream)
chives to garnish

Preparation
Cut the squash in half lengthways and remove the seeds and peel away the thick skin.

Chop into small pieces.

Place in a large saucepan with the celery, onions and garlic and dry-fry over a low heat for 2-3 minutes.

Add the thyme, stock and bay and simmer gently until the vegetables are soft.

Remove the bay leaves and liquidise soup in blender until smooth.

Return the soup to the pan, adjust the consistency with a little extra stock if required and season with salt and black pepper.

Just before serving, remove from the heat and stir in the fromage frais. Divide into serving bowls. Serve the butternut squash soup with a swirl of fromage frais and a pinch of finely chopped chives.

Jill's Multi-Purpose Dressing

Tools
Small bowl

Ingredients
4 tbsp. olive oil
5 tbsp. balsamic vinegar
1-2 cloves pressed garlic
¼ tsp. dijon mustard
1 handful fresh cilantro chopped (optional)
Salt and pepper (to taste)

Preparation
Mix ingredients into bowl and stir
Serve on any salad and enjoy!

Spinach and Strawberry Salad

Strawberries are a great way to jazz up your greens with both flavour and colour. The heart-shaped silhouette of the strawberry is the first clue that this fruit is good for you. These potent little packages help protect your heart, and keep the immune system strong. They are among the top 20 fruits in antioxidant capacity. Need I say more? Enjoy this salad as a side dish or add a veggie burger, organic chicken or fish and have it as a meal.

Tools
Large Bowl

Ingredients
6 cups baby spinach
1 pint fresh strawberries, wash, hull and slice
¼ cup thinly diced red onion
¼ cup walnut pieces or almond slices, lightly toasted

Optional
1 cup cooked quinoa

Preparation
In a large bowl combine the spinach, onion, strawberries and nuts.

Pour dressing over salad (see recipe below) toss well to combine.

Spinach and Strawberry Salad Dressing

Tools
Small bowl

Ingredients
2 tbsp. balsamic vinegar
½ tsp. dijon mustard
4 tbsp. extra virgin olive oil
salt and freshly ground pepper, to taste

Preparation
In a small bowl, whisk together the balsamic and mustard

Slowly whisk the olive oil until well combined

Season with salt and freshly ground pepper

Roasted Broccoli "Super" Salad

Superfoods are nutrient powerhouses that contain large doses of antioxidants, vitamins, and minerals. Our bushy green friend, the broccoli, genuinely deserves this status thanks to a full range of nutrients that help keep the body strong and healthy. With all this goodness, it's a super addition to your weekday dinners and perfect for lunch the following day.

Tools
Large bowl
Large baking sheet

Ingredients
12 ounces broccoli crowns, trimmed and cut into bite-size florets (about 4 cups)
1 cup grape tomatoes
1 tbsp extra-virgin olive oil
2 cloves garlic, minced
¼ tsp. salt
½ tsp. freshly grated lemon zest
1 tbsp. fresh lemon juice
10 pitted black olives, sliced
1 tsp. dried oregano

Preparation
Toss broccoli, tomatoes, oil, garlic and salt in a large bowl and mix until evenly coated.

Spread mix evenly on baking sheet.

Heat oven to 450°F and bake until the broccoli begins to brown (about 10 to 13 minutes)

Combine lemon zest and juice, olives and oregano in a large bowl and mix.

Add the roasted vegetables.

Stir to combine.

Serve warm with quinoa, veggie burger, organic chicken or fish.

Steamed Brussels Sprouts with Tahini Dressing

The brussel sprout is one of the most underrated and under-eaten vegetable, full of nutrients and vitamins we should embrace these little green warriors as a yummy side dish. They provide so many health benefits and are a quick and low maintenance dinner option, the trick is in how you cook them.

One of the most nutritious ways of preparing brussels sprouts is to steam them for no more than 5-10 minutes. If you cook them for too long you risk losing a lot of the beneficial nutrients they contain. In addition, if you cook them for too long they will start to have a pungent sulfurous odour, which isn't very nice. In fact, often times when people don't like Brussels sprouts it is because they have only consumed them when they were overcooked.

Tools
Steamer
Medium bowl

Ingredients
1 lb brussels sprouts
2 tbsp. slivered almonds

Preparation
Put 2 inches of water in the bottom of steamer and bring to a boil

Peel off any yellowing leaves from the brussels sprouts and cut into quarters

Put the Brussels sprouts into the steamer and steam for 5 minutes.

Put the Brussels sprouts in a bowl and toss with dressing (see recipe below)

Transfer to medium bowl and toss with dressing and slivered almonds

Tahini Dressing

Tools
Jar (mason jar works well)

Ingredients
¼ cup tahini
¼ cup water
1/8 cup fresh squeezed lemon juice
1 small clove of garlic crushed
1 tbsp. honey
2 pinches of salt (optional)

Combine ingredients into jar and shake well
Add to brussels sprouts mixture

Warm Pesto Root Veggie

This recipe is all about getting back to our "roots". A hearty simple dish that can be a lovely side or a delicious main course served with a veggie burger, grilled organic chicken or fish.

Tools
Roasting pan
Large bowl

Ingredients
3 parsnips, sliced
2 red onions, sliced
2 red peppers, sliced
1 small butternut squash, sliced
2 tbsp olive oil
4 tbsp basil pesto
2 cups or 100 grams mixed greens or spinach leaves
2 tbsp toasted pine nuts
1 garlic clove, crushed

Preparation
Rub the sliced vegetables with olive oil, garlic (salt and pepper to taste)

Place in roasting pan and spread evenly

Heat oven to 350°F and place pan inside for 30 - 40 mins or until golden and soft.

Allow to cool slightly and then put into large mixing bowl.

Mix with basil pesto, greens, and toasted pine nuts.

Serve and enjoy

*To roast squash it is easier to cut in half and deseed, cook face down in a bit of water

WHAT IS QUINOA?
Quinoa is pronounced as keen-wa. Though not technically a grain, quinoa can substitute for nearly any grain in cooking. Actually the seed of a leafy plant, quinoa's relatives include spinach, beets and Swiss chard. It is rich in protein, iron, potassium and other vitamins and minerals, as well as a good source of dietary fibre and is easily digested.

Quinoa Salad

Tools
Medium pot
Large bowl

Ingredients
1 cup cooked quinoa
2 cups mixed greens
1 grilled red pepper
1 grilled zucchini
1 grilled portobello mushroom
10 grape seed tomatoes cut in half
2 spring onions chopped
parsley to taste

DRESSING
1/3 cup balsamic vinegar
1 tbsp olive oil
1 tbsp dijon mustard
1 garlic clove minced
salt & pepper to taste

Preparation
Vegetables can be grilled on the bbq or roasted in the oven.

If roasted mix 1 tsp. olive oil and 1 tbsp balsamic vinegar and pour over vegetables before roasting.

Roast or bbq until lightly brown.

Once vegetables are cooked cut into bite size pieces and mix all above ingredients in a salad bowl. Drizzle dressing and toss.

Quinoa-Veggie Burger, Organic Chicken or Fish is a nice addition to the salad for added protein.

Quinoa Veggie Burger

More and more, people are realizing that going meatless even once or twice a week can have real health benefits, including weight loss and reduced risk of heart disease. Plant-based foods, such as vegetables, beans and lentils, are low in saturated fat and full of fibre, which helps you feel satisfied on fewer calories. Substituting a meat-free meal into your weekly menu is a delicious way to incorporate more vegetables, beans and whole grains into your diet. On your usual burger night why not try this yummy veggie option served with a fresh green salad.

Tools
Medium pot
Large bowl
Frying pan

Ingredients
½ cup uncooked quinoa (results in 2 cups cooked)
1 tsp. oil
1 cup cremini mushrooms, coarsely grated
1 cup coarsely grated zucchini
¾ cup coarsely grated carrot
1 small shallot, minced
1 garlic clove, minced
1 egg, beaten
3 tbsp cornstarch
¼ tsp. salt
1/8 tsp. cayenne pepper

Preparation
Cook quinoa according to package directions, omitting salt, about 14 minutes.

Transfer to a large bowl.

Heat a large, wide frying pan over medium. Add oil, then mushrooms, zucchini, carrot, shallot and garlic. Cook until soft, about 5 minutes.

Add to quinoa. Stir in egg, cornstarch, salt and cayenne.

Heat the same frying pan over medium. Firmly press ½ Cup quinoa mixture into a measuring Cup. Turn and release into pan. Gently press to shape into a patty about 4 inches wide.

Cook until golden and warmed through, about 4 minutes per side. This can also be cooked on the bbq just lightly grill prior. Top with tahini sauce and roasted plum tomatoes.

Cauliflower Rice Burrito Bowl

In trying to get creative with meals while sticking to the veggie theme, try cauliflower rice as a dinner side dish alternative. If you make a big batch you can freeze it making dinner-time a little quicker! Packed with rich nutrients, cauliflower or cabbage flower is one of the commonly used flower-vegetables.

This is a fun dish the family will enjoy and is great for lunch the next day.

Tools
Box grater
Large skillet

Ingredients
2 tbsp grape seed or olive oil
1 head cauliflower, grated
1 lime, juiced
1 tbsp chili powder
2 tsp. onion powder
¾ tsp. salt

Preparation for Cauliflower Rice

Remove the green stems off the cauliflower and chop the head of cauliflower in half.

Grate the whole head (one half at a time) on the box grater. It's okay if you leave some small florets.

In a large skillet, heat oil to medium-high heat. Add the cauliflower, lime juice, chili powder, onion powder, and salt. Stir everything together and cover the skillet.

Cook the cauliflower, stirring consistently, until it is softened and browned, about 15 to 20 minutes.

GUACAMOLE INGREDIENTS
2 ripe avocadoes
2 cloves garlic, minced
1 lime, juiced

2 tbsp red onion, chopped
1 jalapeno, seeded and chopped (optional)
1 roma tomato, seeded and diced
1 tbsp fresh cilantro, chopped
Salt to taste

Preparation for Guacamole
Peel and pit the avocados and place them in a bowl.

Add the lime juice, garlic, onion, jalapeno, and mash with a fork or chop with a knife (to leave the guacamole chunky, use a knife to chop everything together).

Add the chopped tomato and cilantro and mix into the guacamole.

COMBINE CAULIFLOWER RICE AND GUACAMOLE FOR BURRITO BOWLS
1 14-ounce can garbanzo beans
Guacamole
Cauliflower Rice
Pico de Gallo (fresh salsa)
Cilantro for serving

Preparation
Add the garbanzo beans to a saucepan and heat on medium to medium-high until hot.

Dish desired amount of cauliflower rice, and beans into a bowl. Add pico de gallo (salsa) and guacamole and go to town!

The Nutrition Bowl

This is a hearty dish perfect for the fall and there will be leftovers to enjoy for lunch the following day. Tofu is the protein source for this recipe, but feel free to substitute with veggie burger, organic chicken or fish. It's also delish all by itself.

Tools
Medium pot
Skillet
Blender

Ingredients
4 cups brown rice
1 cup beets, grated
1 cup carrots, grated
1 cup purple cabbage, grated
1 cup almonds, toasted
2 cups spinach
1 package firm tofu cut into ½ -inch cubes

Dressing
1/3 cup nutritional Yeast Flakes
2 tbsp water
3 tbsp tamari or soy sauce
3 tbsp apple cider vinegar
1 clove garlic, crushed
¾ cup sunflower oil
1 tbsp tahini paste

Preparation:
Prepare rice and set aside

Sauté tofu cubes in a skillet with a little vegetable oil.

To prepare dressing combine nutritional yeast flakes, water, tamari or soy sauce, apple cider vinegar, tahini and crushed garlic in blender.

Add oil in a steady stream.

To assemble the bowls, place cooked brown rice into 4 bowls, top with beets, carrots, cabbage, spinach leaves, almonds, and sautéed tofu cubes.

Drizzle bowls with the dressing.

White Kidney Bean Mash Up

Beans are a great vegetarian option. They supply important nutrients your body needs. Beans offer complex carbohydrates, protein, important vitamins and minerals, and fibre in every low-fat, cholesterol-free bite. Now that's power-packed nutrition! Thanks to their high fibre and water content, beans are extremely filling; it doesn't take much to feel satisfied. Taking a long time to digest, beans help keep hunger at bay for longer, which means less snacking later.

ARE YOU AFRAID OF BEANS?

Don't be afraid of beans. Once you understand the cause of gas, it's fairly easy to remedy. Beans contain a sugar called oligosaccharide and we lack the enzyme required to break the sugar down. When the sugar arrives in your lower intestinal tract intact, it ferments, creating a build-up of gas. The gas isn't absorbed into the intestine, so the body expels it, creating musical sounds.

The answer to this problem is pretty simple. Cook your own beans rather than using canned, soaking them thoroughly first to allow the sugar to leach out. To avoid having it re-absorbed into the beans, it's a good idea to change the soaking water a few times.

Cooking the beans slowly also makes a difference. A bag of dry beans, once cooked, provides healthful food for many meals and costs less per serving than many other sources of protein. You will love this recipe, no one will guess that it's not mashed potatoes!

Tools
Frying pan
Blender

Ingredients
1 can white kidney beans (drained and rinsed) or 2 cups of cooked dry beans.
salt and pepper to taste
1 clove crushed garlic
dash of butter
¼ cup water (depending on if you like thick or more liquid mash)

Preparation
In a frying pan on medium heat, pour kidney beans and add salt, pepper, garlic and butter.

Once warm, pour all ingredients into a blender adding the water and blend till smooth, place back into pan and heat for serving.

Ratatouille

As cooler weather is approaching we start to crave warm cozy comfort food, why not end the day with a hearty Ratatouille? This is one of my favourite recipes and there's always leftovers to enjoy the next day. This is a nice vegetarian meal.

Tools
Large saucepan

Ingredients
2 aubergines (eggplant)
2 medium carrots (peeled)
1 red pepper
1 yellow pepper
4 zucchinis
4 tbsp olive oil
2 onions
3 garlic cloves - finely chopped
1 tbsp red wine vinegar
1 tsp. crushed fennel seeds
fresh basil to taste
2 cans chopped tomatoes
pepper to taste

Preparation
Slice carrots, aubergines, zucchinis and peppers into hearty size pieces (1 inch) and set aside.

In a large saucepan over medium heat, sauté onion, carrots and garlic in olive oil until tender.

Add the red wine vinegar, crushed fennel seeds, as well as remaining cut veggies along with the canned tomatoes.

Bring to a boil and then lower heat and simmer for 15 minutes. Toss the fresh basil in for the last 5 minutes and stir.

Serve over quinoa, brown rice, or fresh greens. Fast, hearty and healthy!

Spaghetti "sans" Spaghetti

If you are trying to eat less carbs or up your intake of veggies, you need to try spaghetti squash. The flesh of this squash has a firm and stringy consistency so it holds up nicely when mixed with tomatoes, roasted veggies and pesto. Plus a cup of spaghetti squash contains only 10 grams of carbs, compared to 43 grams of carbs found in traditional spaghetti. It is also a low caloric food; one Cup contains only 42 calories, whereas, the spaghetti pasta has 221 calories per Cup.

When baked, spaghetti squash shreds into thin, stringy pieces that work great as a pasta substitute. Serve it hot or cold and dress it with your favourite sauce or simply on its own with a little salt and pepper. Don't let spaghetti squash's size intimidate you - the toughest part will be cutting it in half!

Tools
Large baking dish
Frying pan

Ingredients:
1 spaghetti squash - cut in 4 cubes

For the sauce:
1 tbsp olive oil
1 tbsp rosemary & thyme (or use whatever spices you enjoy in your sauce)
2 garlic cloves crushed
1 onion chopped
1 zucchini chopped
1 red pepper chopped
1 jar of tomato sauce (or make from scratch)

Preparation
Preheat oven at 350° F.

Cut squash in half and take out seeds, place the squash halves in a large baking dish (lined with foil for easy clean up) cut side up.

Sprinkle salt and pepper evenly over both halves and drizzle lightly with olive oil.

Bake until tender and so skin can easily be pulled away from the flesh, about 1 hour.

While the squash is baking, in a frying pan add oil, onions, vegetables and garlic and cook on medium heat until soft, then add tomato sauce and simmer for 20 minutes.

Place squash on serving plate, add sauce, and spaghetti night is served!

Mediterranean Burger

Tools
Mixing bowl
Frying pan

Ingredients
¼ cup (1 ounce) crumbled light feta cheese (optional)
$1/3$ cup oats
1 tbsp. minced red onion
2 tbsp. Worcestershire sauce
2 tbsp. chopped fresh basil
2 tbsp. chopped fresh oregano
1 pinch of Salt
¼ tsp. freshly ground black pepper
1 lb lean ground turkey (substitute with Black Beans for vegetarian)
1 garlic clove, minced
olive oil for brushing
2 (6-inch) whole-wheat pitas, toasted and halved

Preparation
In a mixing bowl combine all ingredients and mix well.

Form into 4 patties and brush lightly with oil.

Cook on bbq or frying pan.

Toast pita and serve open faced with toppings such as grilled red peppers, tomatoes, lettuce and avocado.

This is also a great recipe to make in advance. Freeze burgers for a quick, ready to eat meal.

Banana Bread

Enjoying baked goods while sticking to a low-fat nutritious plan can present a challenge. But making your own breads, muffins and cookies at home allows you to control the amount of fat in the recipe. Replacing the oil in baked goods with unsweetened applesauce reduces the fat content of your recipe, adds moisture and additional sweetness to the finished product. Enjoy!

Tools
Large bowl
Loaf pan

Ingredients
4 super ripe bananas
2 cups all-purpose flour (can substitute with whole wheat or buckwheat flour)
1 cup white sugar
1 tsp. vanilla extract
1 tsp. baking soda
1 tsp. baking powder
½ tsp. cinnamon
2 eggs
½ cup unsweetened applesauce

Preparation
Mash bananas in a bowl.

Add all other ingredients and mix well.

Pour into loaf pan (grease if necessary).

Bake at 350 degrees F for 50 to 60 minutes, or until toothpick inserted into center of cake comes out clean.

Avocado Chocolate Pudding

Tools
Blender

Ingredients

2 medium sized, ripe avocados
7 - 9 fresh dates, pitted and roughly chopped
1¼ cups coconut milk, almond milk, or filtered water
1/3 cup raw cacao powder, or more to taste
1 tsp. natural vanilla extract or pure vanilla bean powder
1 pinch of unrefined sea salt

Preparation
Soak the dates in milk or water for 10 to 30 minutes.

In a blender, place the avocado flesh, dates (along with their soaking milk or water), cacao powder, vanilla, and salt. Blend until smooth.

You may need to add a little more liquid to facilitate blending. Scrape the sides of the blender down a few times during the process. Adjust ingredients to taste.

Transfer into serving dishes and put in fridge for 1 hour. Garnish with your choice of toppings, such as dried coconut, grated dark chocolate, or berries.

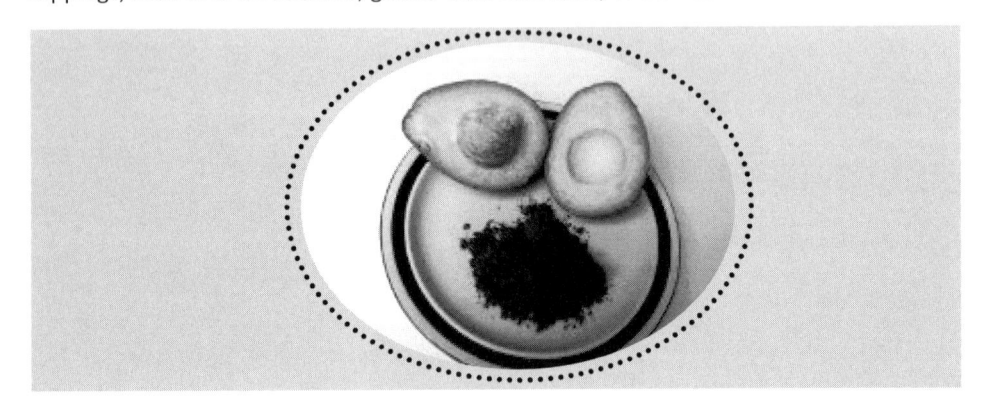

Chapter 10

Toxins and Chemicals Everywhere?

My journey through the last five years has been one of incredible learning and growth, but it has also been full of shock, disappointment and disbelief at the toxins and chemicals in our world. After a diagnosis of skin cancer I started questioning all the products I had been applying to my body and using in my home. It sparked a thirst for information and a passion to bring awareness to others. With so many hidden toxins in our daily products, it takes work to stay healthy. This work is crucial. But, it's not easy....

I was a creature of habit when it came to my beauty products. Shampoo, crème rinse, mousse, and hair spray to make my hair silky smooth, body soap that lathered beautifully making my skin so soft, and body crème that was so creamy and felt so amazing that I reapplied morning and night.

To my surprise and horror, most of my products were rated between 6 and 8 on the Environmental Working Group (www.ewg.com) website, which was highly toxic. This company researches and rates various products on a scale of 0-10. Where a rate of 0 is the best choice, and 10 would be the worst choice. The great thing about this company is they list the ingredients and tell you what the potential health hazards may be. Every time you look up a product, you will be a more educated consumer. You will start to notice that a lot of the same toxins appear regularly in the products.

I don't think I ever really thought about the fact that everything I put on my skin went right into my body. Until something like cancer happens, there is this assumption that all products must be fine or they wouldn't be in the store. Now, I know better.

I threw out hundreds of dollars' worth of products in the first few weeks after diagnosis. Sitting at my computer checking each label from my beauty products and getting more and more upset at what I didn't know.

Knowledge is power and the gift of cancer brought me large amounts of knowledge, frustration and sadness. All I wanted to do was look good and healthy, but applying a number of toxins on my body every day was not achieving that.

Do you know how many toxins you wear every day? For women, in particular, you can be wearing hundreds of toxins just in the beauty products you use each day. Each item in our daily routine can have more than 10 toxins or chemicals within the ingredients list. If you multiply that by the number of products you use every day, it can really add up. Some of these chemicals can stay in the body for days and wreak havoc with our hormones.

Below I have compiled a list of the regularly used chemicals and details to help you identify the concerns. The list is daunting, no question, but it's meant as a quick reference guide to understand what some of the ingredients in your product may be linked to.

BEAUTY PRODUCT TOXINS

ALUMINUM Used as an active ingredient in antiperspirants to stop the flow of sweat. It blocks the sweat duct so you don't smell. Studies show traces of aluminum have been found in breast cancer tumours. There are many deodorants available now that are "aluminum free"	FOUND IN: Deodorant/antiperspirant LABELLED AS: Aluminum POTENTIAL HEALTH CONCERNS Breast cancer, Alzheimer's disease, Parkinson's disease
BUTYLATED HYDROXYANISOLE (BHA) & BUTYLATED HYDROXYTOLUENE (BHT) Preservative used in beauty products and food products *International Agency for Research on Cancer:* Possible Human Carcinogen *Health Canada:* High Human Health Priority	FOUND IN: Lipstick, cosmetics, cereals, crackers, meats, sausage LABELLED AS: BHA, BHT POTENTIAL HEALTH CONCERNS: Endocrine or hormone disruptor, allergies, liver, thyroid and kidney disorders

DIETHANOLAMINE/DEA: Used to make cosmetics smooth and creamy	FOUND IN: Moisturizer, sunscreen LABELLED AS: DEA POTENTIAL HEALTH CONCERNS Liver cancer, skin and thyroid issues
FORMALDEHYDE Formaldehyde is a preservative used in a variety of products. FDA identifies it as a carcinogen	FOUND IN: Manufacturing products, plastics, insecticides, building materials, textiles/clothing, cosmetics, personal care, cleaning products, keratin hair, laundry soap LABELLED AS: Formaldehyde, Methanal, Methyl Aldehyde, Methylene Glycol, Methylene Oxide POTENTIAL HEALTH CONCERNS: Potential increase risk of cancer and respiratory issues, allergic reaction, headache, behaviour changes, skin irritation
LEAD Used for colouring in a variety of products. Recent studies have found high levels of this toxic heavy metal in lipstick. Linked to brain and blood disorders and can potentially interfere with fetal development in pregnant women. Cosmetics can also contain other metals such as Mercury, Aluminum, Cadmium, Chromium and Manganese so look for organic products whenever possible	FOUND IN: Lipstick, eye makeup, fossil fuels, paint, batteries, toys LABELLED AS: Lead POTENTIAL HEALTH CONCERNS Brain, blood, fetal development, behavioural issues

NITROSAMINES Chemical compound used in the manufacturing process of beauty, pesticide and tobacco products. Nitrites are used as a preservative, colouring and flavouring in food such as bacon, lunch meats, hot dogs and other foods. Frying, grilling at high temperatures cause nitrates and amines to produce nitrosamines. According to Safecosmetics.org, Nitrosamines are "banned/found unsafe for use in cosmetics in Canada" International Agency for Research on Cancer identifies this as Possible Human Carcinogen	FOUND IN: Manufacturing, cosmetics, pesticides, rubber products, tobacco, e-cigarettes, food products LABELLED AS: Sodium Nitrite/Nitrate, DEA and TEA POTENTIAL HEALTH CONCERNS: Cancer, Alzheimer's, Type 2 Diabetes, Liver disorders
PARABENS A preservative used in everything from shampoo to toothpaste. Research shows parabens can mimic how hormones act in the body, therefore potentially causing hormonal imbalances. They have also been linked to breast cancer.	FOUND IN: Shampoo, Lotion, Toothpaste LABELLED AS: Methylparaben, Butylparaben, Ethylparaben, Propylparaben POTENTIAL HEALTH CONCERNS Estrogenic, mimic hormones, link to Breast Cancer

PER FLUORINATED CHEMICALS Used in non-stick products and stain resistant in materials	FOUND IN: Non-stick pans, furniture, carpets, clothing, fast food wrappers LABELLED AS: PFC's POTENTIAL HEALTH CONCERNS Linked to cancer, mimic hormones leading to hormonal imbalance
PHTHALATES/FRAGRANCE Phthalates are chemicals used to soften plastics and retain scent. Note: There are no regulations that require the ingredients of added scents or "fragrance" to be disclosed. They are considered "trade secrets." So if something smells great, check it out at the Environmental Working Group's website www.ewg.com.	FOUND IN: Personal care products like perfume, hair spray, nail polish, laundry products, used to carry the scent, pharmaceuticals, medical devices, children's toys and IV bags/tubes LABELLED AS: Phthalates, fragrance, Diethyl Phthalate, Dibuty Phthalate, Di(2-ethylhexyl) phthalate (DEHP) POTENTIAL HEALTH CONCERNS: Mimic hormones, link to problems with liver, kidney, reproductive organs, increase risk of cancer, birth defects, asthma

PROPYLENE GLYCOL AND POLYETHYLENE GLYCOL: Used as a solvent for industrial and beauty products to prevent products from drying out. Material Safety Data Sheet published by National Institute for Occupational Health and Safety urges workers to avoid skin contact with this toxic chemical	**FOUND IN:** Industrial antifreeze, brake/hydraulic fluid, paint, airplane de-icer, facial, hand and body moisturizers, deodorant **LABELLED AS:** Propylene Glycol, PG, Polyethylene Glycol, PEG **POTENTIAL HEALTH CONCERNS** Neurotoxin linked to Dermatitis, Kidney damage and liver abnormalities in scientific and animal testing, allergic reactions
SODIUM LAURYL SULFATE OR SODIUM LAURETH SULFATE: Used as a foaming agent in industrial cleaning and beauty products According to American College of Toxicology: "SLS can stay in the body for up to 5 days accumulating in the heart, liver, lungs and brain."	**FOUND IN:** Engine degreaser, garage/concrete floor cleaner, car wash soap, shampoo, toothpaste **LABELLED AS:** Sodium Lauryl Sulfate, Sodium Laureth Sulfate, SLS **POTENTIAL HEALTH CONCERNS:** Skin, eye and respiratory irritation, toxic to aquatic life
TOLUENE A petrochemical solvent used in nail polish, gasoline, paints, fragrance. Smells like paint thinner.	**FOUND IN:** Nail polish, solvents to dissolve paints, sealants **LABELLED AS:** Toluene, Methylbenzene, Toluol **POTENTIAL HEALTH CONCERNS:** Headaches, dizziness, nausea, reproductive issues

TRICLOSAN Antibacterial and antifungal product used in beauty and cleaning products. Used to prevent growth of bacteria, mold and mildew. This has also been identified as a hormone disrupter. *Environmental Protection Agency* classifies Triclosan "as a pesticide stating it poses a risk to both human health and the environment" *Health Canada* – Identified on the Cosmetic Ingredient "hotlist", a list detailing ingredients that are either prohibited or restricted for use in Canada. *FDA* – Due to health concerns they are continuing with further scientific testing	FOUND IN: Hand Sanitizer, soap, mouth wash, toothpaste, deodorant LABELLED AS: Triclosan, Lexol300, Microban, Biofresh POTENTIAL HEALTH CONCERNS: Endocrine or hormone disruptor, weakens immune system, potential cause of cancer

After learning about all the toxins, the next challenge was finding products that I could trust, but that also worked well. This was not an easy process.

Skincare was, without a doubt, the most difficult. Many of the natural products are hard to rub into the skin, unlike mainstream products that have chemicals to make them smooth and creamy. Sunscreen was brutal to replace. It rubs on thick and white. I looked like a ghost! So, for a few years I just preferred to stay covered up.

Trying different products eventually led me to the ones I now use, which I've shared below. Over the years I have found that I actually use products less frequently, but my skin definitely looks better and younger now. How can that be? I'm a perfect example that beauty products aren't what make your skin healthy; it's what you put in your body.

BEAUTY PRODUCTS I CURRENTLY USE

I've listed below some fabulous products I've found over the years and the companies that make them. All the ingredients are listed, nothing hidden. It's not easy to find products without a little bit of preservative to extend the life of the product, but there is no need to have your products laden with toxic chemicals.

Coconut oil is excellent for the skin and can be applied topically. Of course, a great option is to make your own products and I've identified a few below, but when time doesn't allow for that, here are some great options.

TEETH/ORAL CARE	Product Name: Living Libations, Haliburton, Ontario Toothpaste –Neem Enamelizer Ingredients: Neem, cinnamon, coconut oil, saponified olive oil, sodium bicarbonate, and spring water
TEETH/ORAL CARE	Product Name: Living Libations, Haliburton, Ontario Healthy Gum Drops Ingredients: Super-critical extracts and essences of seabuckthorn berry, rose otto, oregano, peppermint, clove, tea tree, cinnamon, and thyme linalool. Also, Anti-bacterial and anti-fungal
HAIR	Product Name: Eli's Organic Black Shampoo Ingredients: Aqua, Plantain Skin , Cocoa Pod, Palm Kernel Oil or Coconut Oil, Shea Butter, Vegetable Glycerine, Castor Oil, Camomile

HAIR	Product Name: Eli's Organic Leave in Conditioner Ingredients: Distilled aqua, oat flakes, black castor oil, moringa oil, argan oil, vegetable glycerin, grape seed and baobab essential oil.
FACE	Product Name: Eli's Spot Remover Night Crème Ingredients: Aqua, shea butter, oat flakes, grapefruit oil, lime, multifruit, baobab, & cucumber.
FACE	Product Name: Margc Cherry Vitamin C Face Ingredients: Homemade Coconut Oil, Vitamin C Serum, Vitamin C Ester, Orange Peel Butter, Avocado Butter, Yucca Root Powder, Rice, Powder, Almond Oil, Orange Peel Oil, Vitamin E Oil, Neem Oil, Willow Bark Extract, Raspberry Extract, Tocopherol Pam Stearic Acid, Emulsifying Wax, Xanthum Gum, Polysoccharide Gum, Green Clay, Citric Acid, and Rice Alcohol.
BODY	Product Name: Artisana Ingredients: Raw, Organic, Extra Virgin Coconut Oil You can eat it, use it on face, body, hair, it doesn't get more natural than this

BODY	Product Name: Nutiva *When choosing a coconut oil, be sure to look for: cold pressed, unrefined, organic, and raw. Now that the benefits of coconut oil is in the news there are lots of not so great one's on the market. Ingredients: Organic, Extra Virgin Coconut Oil
BODY	Product Name: Nature's Aid Skin Gel This is an incredibly versatile product. With only 5 ingredients, it's very healing. According to the bottle, Nature's Aid is "effective for first aid, prevent spread of infection, speeds cell regeneration, gives skin a more youthful appearance, soothes irritation from cancer treatment" Ingredients: Aloe Vera, Vitamin E, Witch Hazel, Rosemary, Tea Tree

BODY	Product Name: Living Libations, Seabuckthorn All Over Body Lotion Ingredients: Spring water, jojoba, tamanu, organic herbal infusions of seabuckthorn berries, marsh mallow root, slippery elm, chamomile, chickweed, rose hips; seaweed extract; aloe vera; acacia; essential oils of lavender, vetiver grapefruit, palmarosa; supercritical antioxidants of sage and rosemary.
BODY	Product Name: Eli's Body Shop, Ghana, Eli's Black Soap Ingredients: Plantain Skin, Cocoa Pod, Palm Kernel Oil or Coconut Oil, Shea Butter, Olive Oil, Vegetable Glycerine
BODY	Product Name: Eli's Body Shop, Ghana, Eli's Shea+Coca+Olive Body Oil Ingredients: Shea butter (inherent vitamins A, E, & F), cocoa butter, shea oil, olive oil, baobab oil, and cocoa aroma

Body	Product Name: Margc Cherry/, Chicago, Souffle Body Crème Ingredients: Homemade Coconut Oil, Turmeric Powder, Cocoa Butter, Avocado Butter, Shea Butter, Flax Seed Oil, Jojoba Oil, Yucca Root Powder, Rice Powder, Tapioca Powder, Honey Powder, Aloe, Jelly, Lavender Oil, Sweet Orange Oil, Rose Seed Oil, Neem Oil, Sesame Oil, Grape Seed Oil, Aloe Vera Oil, Leaf Extract, Soy Oil, Cider Wood Oil, Vitamin AB from Carrot Oil, Wheat Germ Oil, Licorice Extract, Marigold Flower Extract, Horse Chestnut Extract, Turmeric Oil, Asian Beeswax, Carnauba Wax, Rose Water, Distilled Water, Mineral Sea Salt, Alcohol from Rice, Palm Oil, and Lavender

As you can see most of the products have less than 10 recognizable ingredients. Good companies want you to know their ingredients are safe.

The more ingredients you see, the more likely there is to be some form of chemical compound found in the product. This doesn't mean it's horrible. Most good companies will detail what the ingredients are in layman's terms within brackets beside the long formal name.

Eg. Butyrospermum Parkii (Shea Butter)

Just remember we can't always have perfectly pure ingredients, but if we're making a conscious effort to do the best we can, we can reduce our health risks.

Along with my healthy routine of brushing, gum drops, and flossing, I include **Oil pulling** as a daily routine for my teeth. Simply take 1 tbsp. of Organic coconut oil and swish around in the mouth for 10-20 minutes, spit out in the garbage (not down the sink), rinse with salt water and brush your teeth. Then you're good to go.

WHAT ARE THE BENEFITS OF OIL PULLING?

Oil Pulling is an ancient Ayurveda remedy that's been used for thousands of years. When you swish coconut oil around in your mouth it helps "pull out" a variety of bacteria. Your mouth is a haven for lots of toxins. Unless you're flossing after every meal, it's hard to keep up with the bacteria that can accumulate in your mouth. With oil pulling, the bacteria gets stuck in the oil and you spit them out along with the oil.

It's really not that bad. Some people have an issue with gag reflexes, but I've never experienced it. Your mouth will feel amazing after doing this and there are many benefits.

Here are some reported benefits people have experienced:

Reduce harmful bacteria
Prevent Halitosis (bad breath)
Reduced plaque and gingivitis
Improved gum health
Increased energy
Sinus relief
Whiter teeth
Reduced inflammation by removing harmful bacteria
Clearer skin

I do my 10-20 minute rinse routine first thing in the morning while I use my Rebounder/mini trampoline and catch up on the news. Multi-tasking at it's best.

SKIN PROTECTION:

It's been quite the experience for me learning how to protect my skin after years of sun-tanning. The first few years I was afraid to go in the sun at all. I had read all the toxins in sunscreens and actually questioned whether that wouldn't be worse for the skin than the sun. I continued to stay fully clothed when outdoors. Over time I have found natural sunscreens like *Badger* and *Green Beaver* work really well or wearing a surf shirt allows me to enjoy the outdoors without being fearful of a reoccurrence. I do have several moles from years of sun exposure, so I'm very cautious as recommended by my dermatologist.

With the depletion of the Ozone layer our skin needs to be either covered by protective clothing or sunscreen. Educating ourselves on the top chemicals in sunscreen is the first step. Luckily we also have some amazing passionate people at the Environmental Working Group who continually research and let us know what sunscreens are best. Look for their Top sunscreen list each year.

Let's review the top regularly used chemicals in sunscreen:

CHEMICAL: Retinyl Palmitate	Used For: Retinyl Palmitate is not required to protect you from the sun, it is used to help reduce signs of aging. A lab test in mice showed some results (although as yet unpublished by the FDA due to lack of peer review) that are of concern to many dermatologists. The study showed with sunlight this chemical may increase the development of skin tumours. It's being reviewed by the FDA, but I choose not to use it when this is a potential finding. Since it's not required for sunscreen, some companies have stopped including it in their products. Health Concerns: Potentially increases the risk of developing skin tumours and lesions when sunscreen is worn in the presence of sunlight

CHEMICAL: Oxybenzone Also known as benzophenone-3, BP3, Uvinul M40, Eusolex 4360, Escalol 567	Used For: Oxybenzone is a stabilizer. In a 2006 study, it was shown that oxybenzone is potentially carcinogenic and has destructive effects on DNA when exposed to sunlight Again, more information is needed but if Dermatologists have concerns, so do I. Health Concerns: Can act as hormone disruptors. Potentially affects sexual development and reproductive function in children. In girls, this means early sexual development. For boys, it affects the production of testosterone and stunts testicular development.
CHEMICAL: PABA	Used For: UV Filter Health Concerns: May damage DNA and cause genetic mutation when exposed to sunlight. Not used much anymore, but some products may still include it. Can also be listed as padimate-O, octyldimethyl, ethylhexyl dimethyl PABA, EHDP, Escalol 507

Chemical: Methylparaben	Used for: Preservatives Health Concerns: Found in high concentrations in breast cancer tumors and researchers have also found that when exposed to UVB rays, it increases cell death in human skin

Top Household toxic chemicals

Have you ever taken a good look at your household cleaning products and its ingredients? You won't find many or at least very little information to indicate what's actually cleaning your home.

Cancer diagnosis was a difficult journey, but this gift of learning has continued to inspire me for over five years now. For many years, I believed the best cleaning products were the ones that cleaned with very little effort, smelled amazing and left a lingering scent for a few days. I had no idea I was surrounded with toxins that I was choosing to use. We don't have much control over environmental issues and air quality, but it's our choices for the products used in our house.

When I started researching household chemicals, I was blown away to find that I had to really, really dig to find out what was in these products. Even if I did find something, the list was far from complete. Manufacturers don't have to disclose the chemicals/toxins in their products, only the warnings. I changed everything I could and started to make my own cleaning products with only a few great ingredients. Cleaning with products like vinegar, lemon, baking soda and water just like my Mom did on the farm was interesting to me. We've come full circle.

It took lots of trial and error (mixing baking soda and vinegar gave me many bubbles and lots of laughter) and muscle. It takes a little longer to clean this way but it makes me feel good about not only my health, but the environment. Household products contain chemicals that are also harmful to the planet. Our world has advanced so far, but what has it done for us? Sure, toxic products clean faster but the side effects are plenty.

After learning just how many toxins I had in my shopping bag so that my home would be clean and fragrant, I was horrified. Now, my home is just as fragrant with the wonderful scent of lemon. Fresh and clean, just the way it should be.

BELOW IS A LIST OF SOME HIDDEN TOXINS AND WHERE THEY'RE USUALLY FOUND.

TOXIN/CHEMICAL	DESCRIPTION
TOXIN/CHEMICAL Phthalates Phthalates are usually found listed as "Fragrance" and will be found in any product that smells good or "new"	<u>Found In:</u> Air fresheners, laundry soap, dish soap, cleaners <u>Potential Health Risks:</u> Endocrine or hormone disruptors, birth defects and genital development
TOXIN/CHEMICAL 2-Butoxyethanol Used for multiple cleaning purposes	<u>Found In:</u> Window, all-purpose, floor cleaners <u>Potential Health Risks:</u> Liver, kidney, and nerve damage
TOXIN/CHEMICAL Ammonia Used for multiple cleaning purposes	<u>Found In:</u> Window, all-purpose, toilet, drain, oven cleaners and floor wax <u>Potential Health Risks:</u> Allergies, lung/breathing issues such as asthma and chronic bronchitis
TOXIN/CHEMICAL Chlorine Used for multiple cleaning purposes	<u>Found In:</u> Toilet cleaners, shower mildew cleaners, dishwasher detergent, city water to remove bacteria <u>Potential Health Risks:</u> Respiratory, skin, eyes, potential thyroid disruptor

Toxin/Chemical Sodium Hydroxide Used as strong industrial cleaner and a few very strong household products	Found In: Disinfectants, oven cleaner, drain products, stain removers Potential Health Risks: Respiratory, lung, skin, eyes, throat

So now that we know our cleaning products are full of toxins with no disclosure, how can you tell what products are safe to buy? This may sound crazy, but the only way to really gage is by looking at the warning label.

Here are some tips for making your choice:

Danger/Poison = Most Toxic

Warning = Moderately Toxic

Caution = Mildly Toxic

Each of these comments should be followed with instruction for what you need to be careful. The better choice is to look for a product that doesn't have any of these warnings.

Here are some marketing tricks to be aware of as well:

Non-toxic
Natural
Eco-friendly

All these terms mean nothing unless it gives specific information like:

Solvent Free
No Petroleum-based ingredients
No Phosphates
No Chlorine
No Petroleum Products

If you're buying cleaning products from a large manufacturer, remember, they are in business to make money and the cheaper the ingredients they can use, the more profitable the product. Another thing to watch for is if it cleans really easily, it probably has several toxic chemicals in it. Cleaning should require a bit of elbow grease. Be suspicious if you don't see clear labels.

Let's look at some homemade cleaning products and solutions just like what your Granny used to use.

HOME-MADE INGREDIENTS:

Baking Soda	Used For: This is the most versatile product I know of. I've used it for cleaning everything in the kitchen and bath. Also great for teeth whitener in moderation as this can be hard on the enamel. Tea stains in my favourite mug….gone! Try it for a hand, face, body soap too. How To Use It: Simply add ½-1 cup baking soda, water, 10-12 drops of an essential oil and mix it up to paste consistency. Voila, you have a fabulous new soap that cost a lot less than the store bought kind and it's without all those harmful chemicals.

Vinegar	Used for: Cleans windows and mirrors beautifully, cuts grease, removes mildew in the shower, removes stains, odors, clean kitchen counters, faucets, washing machine, coffee maker….basically anything in your house can be cleaned with vinegar. Combine with an essential oil and it will smell great too. How To Use It: 1/2 cup vinegar, ½ cup water, 10-20 drops essential oil of your choice
Olive Oil	Used For: Cleans wood furniture. Add a little lemon to this and you have an instant wood furniture polish with a wonderful fresh scent. How To Use It: Mix 1 cup olive oil and ½ cup fresh lemon juice. Use soft cloth to clean furniture. Test a small area to ensure it works on your furniture. Prepare and use on same day
Lemon	Used For: Glass cleaner, cuts grease, mildew, mold, household bacteria, makes countertops shine! How To Use It: Add ¼ cup of fresh lemon juice and water in a spray bottle

Sea Salt	Used For: Great to add to baking soda to make a scrub for those tougher to clean areas
	How To Use It: When cleaning with baking soda just add a little sea salt to your cloth for extra scouring power.

Essential Oils to use in homemade products

Tea Tree Oil	Benefits: Antifungal, antiseptic, antimicrobial, antiviral, bactericidal, insecticidal
Lemon Oil	Benefits: Antimicrobial, antiseptic, anti-bacterial
Lavender	Benefits: Antiseptic, antifungal, anti-inflammatory, anti-infectious
Peppermint	Benefits: Antiseptic
Eucalyptus	Benefits: Antiseptic
Sweet Orange	Benefits: Antiseptic, antifungal, antibacterial

It's been a long process learning all this information, but it was indeed a gift. I had never looked at any products, beauty or home, with any concern prior to diagnosis. The only thing I cared about was how creamy a moisturizer felt on my skin, how amazing it smelled or how fast I could clean my home. Never once did I think I couldn't trust the products in the stores. I spent hours researching and calling my sister, Sandra, in disbelief as I discovered another toxic product I'd been using. Making my own products feels great and I feel very accomplished. I know what's in them, that it's good for me, and good for the environment.

The root cause of cancer is oxygen deficiency which creates an acidic state in the human body.

Dr. Otto Warbug

Chapter 11

The Exercise and Disease Connection

"Those who can't find time for exercise, will eventually have to make time for illness"

Unknown

We have all heard that exercise is good for us, but do you know the role it has in preventing many serious illnesses including cancer? Until my diagnosis I didn't realize how crucial exercise was to maintaining true health. I didn't understand the most important part of exercise…..Oxygen or the role it plays in the body. Oxygen is vital in the survival of life, but not just from a breathing perspective. Research shows that low levels of oxygen in the blood is a contributing factor to many diseases. According to Nobel Prize winner Dr. Otto Warbug, "the root cause of cancer is oxygen deficiency which creates an acidic state in the human body."

His research also shows that cancer cells are anaerobic, meaning they do not require oxygen, and *cannot survive* in high levels of oxygen achieved by a nutritious diet and daily exercise. Let me repeat that, *cancer cannot survive in high levels of oxygen….*

See the correlation? Chapter 7 talks about the importance of eating a diet consisting of 80% Alkaline and 20% Acid to maintain a healthy Potential Hydrogen (PH) level. This gives even more reason to ensure this is accomplished. Keeping the body's alkaline/acid level balanced is Cancer Prevention 101.

For many years I sat at a desk, like a large percentage of the population, and exercised outside of work hours. I was always committed to my morning routine of 30 minutes run or bike and 20 minutes weight training. It maintained a very "healthy looking" body for many years. However, there were many days and weekends when I would not get up from my desk for 12-14 hours straight.

Of course, there were bathroom breaks but even those were not that frequent as my body adapted to the sedentary work environment. I have to say, looking back, that my body did pretty good with the limited movement it was actually receiving and the acidic food/toxins it was receiving from me daily. Thank god I was at least committed to a morning workout. *Cancer doesn't have to look sick.....*

DANGERS OF SITTING

An Australian study, published in the Archives of Internal Medicine, states that if you sit 11 hours a day or more you have a 40% higher risk of early death. Yes, you read that right....40%. What's a typical day for most people? Sitting during meals, commuting to work and home, watching TV after a long day, computer time, meeting friends after work for a late drink or a bite to eat, and sleeping.

Is this your life? If you're work requires you to be predominantly at a desk, I would guess you are sitting more than 10 hours when you include meals, travel time and work. Think about your day. I didn't recognize sitting as a potential precursor to disease and I'm sure most people don't...

Unfortunately, each generation becomes even more sedentary with the amount of social media and technology readily available right in your hand. The study showed that even if you make the time to exercise 30-60 minutes per day, the dangers are still there.

This was my life. I thought exercising in the morning was all I needed. I still find myself getting pulled into the world of desk and computer for hours when I'm focused on a project. I'm more aware now and try to get up regularly. I make the effort to do work standing at a high table, like I am now as I type this. I do get upset with myself when I realize I've been working on something too long because I know better and I know the stagnation it's causing in my body.

It's the non-movement throughout the day that is wreaking havoc on our bodies. The study included 200,000 people and it was determined that regular movement of 2 minutes every 20 minutes can add years to your life. Just 2 minutes.

That sounds very similar to how people lived 30-40 years ago, right? Exercise/movement was just part of life. Jobs were much more physical and there was a lot less terminal disease...connection? I believe so. Now that technology has changed the way we do everything, it's up to us to make that extra effort to protect our body from the stagnation that happens from sitting.

WHAT ACTUALLY HAPPENS WHEN WE SIT?

Blood circulation slows down with long periods of sitting and since blood transfers oxygen and nutrients to the entire body obviously the body will not be working efficiently. This can contribute to a number of diseases:

CANCER	How Reduced Circulation Contributes: Slowed blood means less oxygen is being transported to the blood cells potentially leading to low oxygen levels and higher fermentation of sugar in the cells. An ideal environment for cancer cells to grow. Cancer loves sugar. Exercise Helps: Oxygenate the cells and release toxins from the body. Cancer cannot live in a high oxygen environment. Removing the overload of toxins is key in cancer prevention.
DIABETES	How Reduced Circulation Contributes: Sitting changes the way our bodies deal with sugar. When you eat, your body breaks down the food into glucose, which is then transported in the blood to other cells. Glucose is an essential fuel but persistently high levels increase your risk of diabetes along with heart disease and cancer. Your pancreas produces the hormone insulin to help get your sugar levels back down to normal. How efficiently your body does that is affected by how physically active you are. Exercise Helps: Regulate sugar levels, increase lean muscle mass and reduce body fat

HEART DISEASE/STROKE	How Reduced Circulation Contributes: Slower blood flow means less heart activity and reduction in enzyme called lipoprotein lipase (LPL) that breaks down blood fats. Higher levels of fats in the blood increase the risk of heart disease

Slower blood flow could result in blood clots

Less oxygen to the brain could result in stroke

Exercise Helps: Increase blood flow thereby increasing circulation to all cells |
| **OBESITY** | How Reduced Circulation Contributes: Obesity is considered a sign of inflammation in the body. Sitting contributes to higher fat and sugar levels, more toxins retained in the body fat

Exercise Helps: Build lean muscle to burn fat, stabilize blood sugar, improve cardiovascular strength, increase metabolism resulting in more efficiently utilizing nutrients |

So without exercise and regular movement, the body simply slows down all processes opening up lots of opportunity for illness to take hold. These are just the potential deadly diseases, but think about all the little miserable flus, colds, fatigue, and immune system problems that could easily be avoided just by keeping the body moving! According to *Statistics Canada*, only 15% of Canadians get the recommended amount of exercise and *Centre for Disease Control* reports that only 20% of Americans get the recommended amount of exercise. Is it surprising that we have high rates of disease? No, and sadly it's getting worse with the continual introduction of new technology.

The blood needs to be constantly flowing to help nourish the body and remove toxins. It's as simple as that. *Stagnation is a precursor to disease* and a healthy lifestyle is key to living a long and happy life. It's really up to you.

You give so much of yourself on a daily basis to others in your life whether it's family, work, friends, or colleagues. Aren't you just as important as everyone else? Unfortunately, a lot of people don't look at it like this. Our society promotes pleasing others, needing to keep everyone happy...what about keeping your body healthy? Where does that fall into your priorities? You're worth 30 minutes a day of exercise and consciously moving every hour. Not only will this help you physically, but will also give you a clear head to accomplish more of your goals, and it might save your life.

Smile and let everyone know that today, you're a lot stronger than you were yesterday

UNKNOWN

I am so much stronger than I was five years ago in so many ways. Cancer was an incredible gift. I've learned that no matter what your circumstances are today, you can learn and grow to be a stronger version of yourself. Strong means so much more than physical strength and exercise provides more than just the external result. Listen to your body and prevent disease.

Exercise is disease prevention for your body. It provides the oxygen that every cell needs to thrive. All these diseases I've mentioned are preventable or kept under control by simply moving the body regularly. Each year there is more and more illness starting at much younger ages. It's time to stop this pattern and take control of your life.

How to incorporate more movement into your day?

1. Drink lots of water.
   As we learned in an earlier chapter, the body requires an average of 8-10 glasses of water per day so if you are drinking this amount you will need to use the bathroom frequently. Use a facility on a different floor or at least a little distance away from your office so you have to walk for 2 minutes.

2. Take the stairs at every opportunity.
   There is always a set right beside the escalator.

3. Walk meetings.
   If you need to meet with a colleague, but don't require a computer or documents this is a fabulous option.

4. Stand while talking on the phone.

5. Invest in a stand-up desk! This is a fantastic option as it can be used either seated or standing just by pushing a button.

6. Set a timer on your phone/computer to remind you it's time to move.

7. Stand on the subway and maybe even hop off a few stops early to walk to your destination.

8. Walk to work.
   I walk every day and it adds up to 20kms each week. It is recommended that we get

10,000 steps per day, but reports show Canadians and Americans only get one third of that requirement.

9. Park away from your destination and walk rather than drive around and around until someone leaves a closer spot.
According to Dr. Mike Evans, the parking spot further away is the one "reserved for people who want to live longer."

10. Dedicated lunch-time walk.
You are worth it and you will be more productive in the afternoon.

EXERCISE CHOICES:

The best exercise is the one you're going to do. Everyone is different and exercise styles vary greatly.

Here are my top choices:

1. Cardio exercise: Walking, running, biking/spin class, aerobic classes, step-mill, and hiking

2. Resistance training: Very important to build/maintain lean muscle mass, especially as we start to age. This is crucial to keep bones strong, prevention of osteoporosis and maintaining a healthy body weight

3. Jump Rope: Did you know that 10 minutes of jump rope is equivalent to 30 min of jogging? Although not easy to jump for 10 minutes, consistency will get you there

4. Team Sports: Great motivator and always tons of fun to be out with friends and meet new ones

5. Rebounding/jumping on mini-trampoline: This is an exercise that I do every day, sometimes 2 times a day for approx 10-20 minutes. This is recognized as an excellent exercise for cancer patients and survivors as it helps stimulate the Lymphatic System, which is so important in the process of detoxification.

6. Stairs. Taking the stairs whenever possible is, of course, a great habit to get into

but you can also do interval sprints on stairs to increase heart rate and work the muscles.

7. Squash or Tennis. Challenge yourself and join a squash ladder or tennis club to have games planned for you. It's a great way to hold you accountable to your exercise commitment.

8. Make Winter your friend too! Skiing, snowboarding, snowshoeing….all great full body workouts with the benefit of fresh air and nature!

9. Yoga: There are many different types of yoga, from Power yoga to a very gentle movement but the one thing they all have in common is mental strength and emotional balancing.

Bottom line: Exercise is crucial for the health of your body and your future. Push yourself to get to your next exercise destination. I promise you will feel so much better after. You won't ever regret "going" to exercise, but you will regret not going.

My Top 10 tips for Healthy Living and Living Stress Free

1. Move! Keep the body in motion. Walk in nature with your feet in the grass. Touching and breathing in Mother Nature helps ground the body. Exercise 30-45 minutes per day incorporating some form of cardio or strength training.

2. Eat a variety of healthy organic foods. Look at food as nourishment and fuel rather than an experiment for your taste buds.

3. Listen to your body. Little signs like aches, twinges, pain, heat, itching, etc. are all ways the body lets you know it needs you to be aware of something.

4. Meditation, Yoga, Tai-Chi
These are all wonderful practices to give your body a reprieve from the world we live in. My practice is my time to give back to my body and thank it for keeping me healthy and happy.

5. Laugh a lot! One of the oldest sayings is still one of the best, "Laughter is the best medicine."

6. Live your life. Don't take life too seriously. Let go of negative thoughts and people. Yes, it really is okay to let go of someone whose energy drains you. We are all on our own journey. Ask yourself why you're hanging on to something or someone if it doesn't feel right?

7. Resist pharmaceutical drugs unless absolutely necessary. Yes, there are definitely times when medical drugs are required, but it's also an easy fix to grab a pill rather than trying to find the underlying cause. If you stay in tune and listen to your body you probably won't need them.

8. Be flexible in your thinking. Life changes, doors close, but the next door that opens is always better.

9. Keep your mind active with things you're passionate about! Passion inspires and creates wonderful positive energy for you and those around you.

10. Always have a goal or trip planned. Creating a vision board at the beginning of each year, or anytime you want, helps to keep you excited and moving forward. This is my annual project every January 1st. It's a great way to start off a new year, by identifying all the things you want to do in the coming year. Open your mind and know that you can do anything you choose!

Chapter 12

Q & A with Dr. Selene Wilkinson, ND

I'd like you to meet Dr. Selene Wilkinson, Naturopathic Doctor and extraordinary woman. Selene helped me change the course of my life and continues to inspire me on a regular basis. She graciously agreed to share her time with me and offer you some of her thoughts on cancer.

What is cancer? In your opinion, what causes it?

Cancer is a group of diseases that involves abnormal cell growth. The cause can be one or a combination of factors such as; genetic predisposition, environmental influences, exposure to toxins, as well as a poor diet and/or lifestyle.

What role can Naturopathic Medicine play in terms of cancer?

Naturopathic Medicine offers an individualized holistic care approach to anyone looking at receiving complementary support alongside their conventional cancer treatments. It consists of diverse treatments such as diet, lifestyle, acupuncture, botanical medicine, supplements, counselling and meditation. Its best role however is in prevention.

What are your dietary recommendations for those with cancer or wanting to do what they can to prevent cancer?

Diet has the potential to help prevent cancer and optimize conventional cancer treatments. Much of our health begins in our stomach and intestines. Most people do not realize that 70% of our immune system lies along the intestinal wall. Therefore maintaining a healthy intestine is extremely important when trying to optimize your health in order for maximum absorption of nutrients.

Plant-based diets have been shown to be important in cancer prevention and treatments. In general, I encourage a diet that can alkalize the body. Sugar, processed foods, meat and dairy products are acidic and should be minimized or avoided. Vegetables, in particular dark green leafy vegetables, create an alkaline environment which is ideal. In addition, I recommend foods that detoxify, boost the immune system and decrease inflammation. Vegetables, fruits and certain components of plant foods, have significant research supporting a protective effect against cancer. Juicing may also be recommended for some patients.

Eating organic food is highly recommended. Pesticides have been linked to cancer and other diseases. If purchasing organic is not always possible due to cost or availability, look at the Dirty Dozen for guidance on which products should be purchased organically - www.ewg.org.

Drinking pure, clean water is extremely important. Starting every morning with a glass of warm water and the juice from half of a fresh organic lemon is recommended to detoxify the body, help with bile production, constipation and alkalize the body. Lemons are acidic, but once ingested they have an alkaline effect on the body.

Obesity also plays a role in the progression and mortality risk of several cancers. Keeping an optimum weight and BMI should be a desired goal for not only general health, but in cancer prevention as well.

Speaking to your primary physician before making any changes to your diet and lifestyle is always recommended.

WHAT LIFESTYLE RECOMMENDATIONS DO YOU SUGGEST FOR PEOPLE?

Lifestyle recommendations are created on an individual bases. Some general suggestions are:

- Live a balanced lifestyle
- Avoid or minimize exposure to toxins
- Eat a balanced diet
- Sleep 7-8 hours a night
- Exercise daily
- Avoid direct contact with the sun during peak hours
- Detoxify
- Daily meditation and deep abdominal breathing

DESCRIBE THE ROLE EMOTIONAL TRAUMA PLAYS IN DISEASE.

Emotional trauma can impact our health greatly. We are just beginning to understand the true depth of the mind-body connection.

In Chinese Medicine each organ is associated with an emotion, for example the lung is associated with sadness. It is very interesting that I often see lung pathologies in patients that have just lost a loved one, or have gone through other life challenges that create sadness.

Studies have shown that one of the most common links in people with longevity is their ability to overcome difficult situations and let go of hardships. Hanging on to grief, guilt, anger, and/or sadness can be detrimental to your health. Working forward through challenging situations using therapy, exercise, journaling, meditation or whatever works for you, is important for both quality and quantity of life.

I recommend yoga, tai chi and/or qigong as they relax the nervous system and reduce stress. Studies show that these types of exercises can be very helpful physically, mentally and emotionally and is therefore important in treatment and prevention of disease.

DO YOU RECOMMEND DETOXIFICATION THERAPIES TO YOUR PATIENTS?

Detoxification may be recommended for some patients, although it is prescribed on a very individualized basis. For some patients I recommend juicing using low glycemic vegetables. For others I recommend botanicals and supplements that can also be used to gently, but effectively support detoxifying organs such as the liver, kidney, skin and lymphatic system. Although it can be an important part of treatment, patients need to be careful as detoxification is very individualized and is suggested only for certain patients, at the appropriate times and using specific methods.

WHAT TREATMENTS DO YOU RECOMMEND FOR YOUR PATIENTS?

Each person requires a tailored treatment plan specifically created for them. There are a number of natural treatments that are used in conjunction with conventional treatments. Some natural treatments may include dietary and lifestyle recommendations, acupuncture, vitamin C IV therapy, supplements, herbs, meditation, exercise therapy and counselling.

Studies show that patients who undergo natural therapies while having chemotherapy and/or radiation have better outcomes. Not only are the side effects more manageable, the outcome of the conventional treatment can be more effective.

WHAT IS THE GREATEST ROADBLOCK TO HEALING?

The stage and type of the cancer is a large factor in healing. The earlier the cancer is detected, and the stronger the persons vitality, the more likely for healing to occur.

HOW CAN FRIENDS AND FAMILY SUPPORT THEIR LOVED ONES WITH CANCER?

Friends and family can help by being a positive and compassionate force in the patient's life. They should be realistic, honest and supportive, both emotionally and physically. Most importantly, listening to the patient and understanding their needs and wishes should be the number one priority.

WHAT DO YOU WISH THAT MORE PEOPLE WITH CANCER KNEW WHEN SEEKING OUT TREATMENTS?

Discussing and evaluating conventional treatment options with ones Medical Doctor is important. In addition, considering supportive alternative treatments from a Naturopathic Doctor that specializes in oncology would be the best course of action.

WHAT ELSE DO YOU WANT PEOPLE TO KNOW ABOUT YOUR WORK WITH DISEASE?

Eat clean, fresh, organic food. Avoid harmful toxins and minimize your exposure to anything that has harsh odour (i.e. new carpet, plastic). Our bodies are designed to process and eliminate toxins through our liver, kidneys, lungs, skin and bowels. If the body is overloaded, disease can occur.

Pay attention and be aware of your thoughts, your actions, and people you surround yourself with. Live in the present, with intention and not in fear.

Everyone should pay attention to their bodies and listen to any messages it may be sending them. See a primary health care physician on regular bases. Assess nutrients and hormones frequently. For example, a vitamin D deficiency is common in Canada and in other parts of the world and is linked to several types of cancers, therefore supplementation is often necessary.

In summary, eat a balanced diet, drink clean water, exercise, sleep 7- 8 hours a night, minimize toxins, detoxify, decrease stress, be around people and do things that make you feel happy and fulfilled.

CERTIFIED FOR IV VITAMIN C INJECTIONS, CAN YOU EXPLAIN WHAT THIS MEANS FOR CANCER PATIENTS?

IV vitamin C injections are gaining attention in playing a supportive role in cancer care. Patients who receive IV vitamin C with other conventional therapies have been shown to improve quality of life, reduce cancer-treatment related symptoms including nausea, fatigue and slow cancer progression.

WHAT ARE YOUR FINAL WORDS OF WISDOM FOR CANCER PATIENTS?

Patients should discuss their treatment options with their Medical Doctor and Naturopathic Doctor, but also do what they can to take care of themselves. Eating well and living a healthy lifestyle can be very empowering and can make a difference.

You can feel Patsy's passion for health and disease prevention throughout the entire book. She offers a great deal of insight and useful resources for anyone looking for ways to optimize their health.

Dr. Selene Wilkinson, ND

Disclaimer for Selene's Q & A chapter:

Information provided is for general information purposes and in no way should be construed as medical advice. Please always remember to contact your healthcare provider to discuss any changes you are considering. Dr. Selene Wilkinson does not assume any liability for the information contained herein.

CONCLUSION - WHAT'S NEXT?

This has been an incredible journey filled with great personal growth, awareness, knowledge and expression. One of the key things I've learned over the past few years is to be open to all experiences and changes. I didn't realize how difficult writing some parts of the book might be or the personal reflection that would be involved. Sometimes, in the moment, frustrations can feel so overwhelming and unfair, but have you ever noticed that when you look back, there was a reason or a lesson that propelled you into another, better, direction? Opportunities present themselves when you are ready. Some of us take a little longer to understand the lesson than others, but in the end things always have a way of working out.

WHERE AM I GOING NOW?

I am quite passionate about health and wellness so I will continue along this path. I'm currently studying to become a Doctor of Naturopathy with a targeted completion of 2016. I'm excited to continue learning and delve even deeper into natural healing techniques. I will also continue to Level II Reiki certification as I believe it is a valuable tool to reduce stress and balance the body. Improving my skills in this area will allow me to continue to share how energy work can promote a healthy lifestyle.

I'm looking forward to speaking for the first time at an international conference in 2015. It's a little intimidating, but also a huge opportunity to share information and, of course, more personal and professional growth. I've also become quite passionate about yoga over the past year, enjoying the benefits it offers the body in so many ways. I will continue to practice and become a yoga instructor one day.

Ultimately, if I was given the opportunity, I would love to host a television show on health and wellness. I believe, interviewing experts on a variety of topics and sharing that information on a public forum could have a huge impact on awareness and disease prevention.

Spending quality time with love ones and quiet time to meditate and journal has special meaning to me since diagnosis. I'm moving toward a simpler life, with less material possessions and more experiences. Travel is definitely in my future. I hope to see and appreciate all the beauty our world has to offer.

I'm open to wherever life takes me. Let the healthy journey continue!

I hope you have enjoyed the book as much as I have enjoyed writing it.

IN MEMORY

I would like to dedicate this book to my cousin Allan Hardiman. Allan, like so many others, did not have the opportunity to learn as I did. Would it have changed his path, no one knows for sure.

Allan's cancer was discovered at a later stage and after an aggressive treatment plan, his journey was sadly cut short. He was diagnosed in March 2012 and left us in Oct 2012. Rest in peace Allan. We miss you.

References

Books

Barnouin, Kim. Skinny Bitch Home, Beauty & Style. Philadelphia: Running, 2011. Print.

Campbell, T. Colin, and Thomas M. Campbell. The China Study: The Most Comprehensive Study of Nutrition Ever Conducted and the Startling Implications for Diet, Weight Loss and Long-term Health. Dallas, Tex.: BenBella, 2005. Print.

Clement, Brian R. Hippocrates Lifeforce: Superior Health and Longevity. Summertown, Tenn.: Healthy Living Publications, 2007. Print.

Colson, Dana G. Your Mouth: The Gateway to a Healthier You : A Yoga-based Approach to Exploring the Connections between Oral Health, Whole Body Wellness and Longevity. Toronto: DJC, 2011. Print.

Crocker, Pat. The Juicing Bible. Pb. ed. Toronto: Robert Rose, 2000. Print.

Emmott, Stephen. Ten Billion. Print.

Fife, Bruce. Oil Pulling Therapy: Detoxifying and Healing the Body through Oral Cleansing. Colorado Springs: Piccadilly, 2008

Gao, Duo. Traditional Chinese Medicine: The Complete Guide to Acupressure, Acupuncture, Chinese Herbal Medicine, Food Cures and Qi Gong. London: Carlton, 2013. Print.

Harper, Harold W., and Michael L. Culbert. How You Can Beat the Killer Diseases. New Rochelle, N.Y.: Arlington House, 1977. Print.

Hm, Anne E., and David J. Hm. Cancer Battle Plan. New York: Jeremy P. Tarcher/Putnam, 1998. Print.

Jensen, Bernard, and Sylvia Bell. Tissue Cleansing through Bowel Management: From the Simple to the Ultimate. 11th ed. Escondido, Calif.: B. Jensen, 1981. Print.

Johnson, Mark. Rapid Raw. Print.

Ratey, John J., and Eric Hagerman. Spark: The Revolutionary New Science of Exercise and the Brain. New York: Little, Brown, 2008. Print.

Shapiro, Debbie. Your Body Speaks Your Mind: Understanding How Your Emotions and Thoughts Affect You Physically. Rev. and Updated ed. London: Piatkus, 2007. Print.

Smith, Jeffrey M. Seeds of Deception: Exposing Industry and Government Lies about the Safety of the Genetically Engineered Foods You're Eating. Fairfield, IA: Yes, 2003. Print.

Tuttle, Will M. The World Peace Diet: Eating for Spiritual Health and Social Harmony. New York: Lantern, 2005. Print.

Wheeler, Virginia, and Edmond G. Addeo. The Conquest of Cancer: Vaccines and Diet. New York: F. Watts, 1984. Print.

Wigmore, Ann. The Hippocrates Diet and Health Program. Wayne, N.J.: Avery Pub. Group, 1984. Print.

Movies

An Inconvenient Truth. Paramount ;, 2007. Film.

Fast Food Nation. 20th Century Fox Home Entertainment, 2007. Film.

Food, Inc. CTV International [ed.] :, 2010. Film.

Forks over Knives. Monica Beach Media :, 2012. Film.

Healing Cancer. Cinema Libre Studio, 2008. Film.

Websites

"American Cancer Society | Information and Resources for Cancer: Breast, Colon, Lung, Prostate, Skin." American Cancer Society | Information and Resources for Cancer: Breast, Colon, Lung, Prostate, Skin. Web. 2014. <http://www.cancer.org/>.

"American College of Toxicology." American College of Toxicology. Web. 2014. <http://actox.org/>.

"RESEARCH. TRANSLATION. PREVENTION." Baker IDI. Web. 2014. <http://www.bakeridi.edu.au/>.

"Select Your Province." - Canadian Cancer Society. Web. 2014. <http://www.cancer.ca/>.

"Canadian Skin Cancer Foundation." Canadian Skin Cancer Foundation. Web. 2014. <http://www.canadianskincancerfoundation.com/

Centers for Disease Control and Prevention. Centers for Disease Control and Prevention, 6 Jan. 2015. Web. 2014. <http://www.cdc.gov/>.

"David Suzuki Foundation." David Suzuki Foundation. Web. 2014. <http://www.davidsuzuki.org/>.

"Energise For Life." Energise For Life. Web. 2014. <http://www.energiseforlife.com/>.

"US Environmental Protection Agency." EPA. Environmental Protection Agency. Web. 2014. <http://www.epa.gov/>.

"Environmental Working Group." Environmental Working Group. Web. 2014. <http://www.ewg.org/>.

"DocMikeEvans." YouTube. YouTube. Web. 2014. <http://www.youtube.com/user/DocMikeEvans>.

"Experience Life." Experience Life. Web. 2014. <https://experiencelife.com/>.

"Home." Green Beaver. Web. 2014. <http://greenbeaver.com/>.

"Greenpeace." Greenpeace. Web. 2014. <http://www.greenpeace.org/usa/en/>.

"Health Canada | Santé Canada." Welcome to the Health Canada Web Site. Web. 2014. <http://www.hc-sc.gc.ca/>.

"Stories That Inspire Us." @healthcentral. Web. 2014. <http://www.healthcentral.com/>.

"Controversial Ingredients to Avoid in Your Personal Care and Beauty Cosmetics." Controversial Ingredients to Avoid in Your Personal Care and Beauty Cosmetics. Web. 2014. <http://www.healthy-communications.com/harmfulingredients1.html>.

"Quotations, Famous Quotes at Quote World." Quotations, Famous Quotes at Quote World. Web. 2014. <http://www.quoteworld.org/>.

"Hippocrates Health Institute | Leading the Field of Natural and Complementary Health Care and Education." Hippocrates Health Institute | Leading the Field of Natural and Complementary Health Care and Education. Web. 2014. <http://hippocratesinst.org/>.

"Huntsman Cancer Institute." Huntsman Cancer Institute. Web. 2014. <http://www.huntsman.com/corporate/a/About us/Social responsibility/Huntsman Cancer Institute>.

"Famous Quotes." BrainyQuote. Xplore. Web. 2014. <http://www.brainyquote.com/>.

Web. 2014. <http://www.iarc.fr/

Web. 2014. <http://www.kidsrighttoknow.com/wp-content/uploads/2014/01/Will-GM-Crops-Feed-the-World-cban-report-summary-2014.pdf>.

"Kris Carr, New York Times Best-selling Author and Wellness Activist." KrisCarrcom RSS. Web. 2014. <http://kriscarr.com/>.

"Front Page." Organic Consumers Association. Web. 2014. <https://www.organicconsumers.org/>.

"Natural Cosmetics and Ayurvedic Skincare Products." Natural Cosmetics and Ayurvedic Skincare Products. Web. 2014. <http://naturalcosmetics.com/>.

"Natural Health News and Scientific Discoveries - NaturalNews.com." NaturalNews. Web. 2014. <http://www.naturalnews.com/>.

Campaign for Safe Cosmetics : Index." Campaign for Safe Cosmetics : Index. Web. 2014. <http://safecosmetics.org/>.

"Healthy Wealthy and Wise | Training and Development." Healthy Wealthy and Wise | Training and Development. Web. 2014. <http://www.healthywealthyandwise.com/>.

"Welcome / Bienvenue." Government of Canada, Statistics Canada. Web. 2014. <http://www.statcan.gc.ca/>.

"The Longevity Now Conference." The Longevity Now Conference. Web. 2014. <http://

www.thelongevitynowconference.com/>.

"U.S. Food and Drug Administration." U S Food and Drug Administration Home Page. Web. 2014. <http://www.fda.gov/

Warburg, Otto, Franz Wind, and Erwin Negelein. "THE METABOLISM OF TUMORS IN THE BODY." The Journal of General Physiology. The Rockefeller University Press. Web. 2014. <http://www.ncbi.nlm.nih.gov/pmc/articles/PMC2140820

"WebMD - Better Information. Better Health." WebMD. WebMD. Web. 2014. <http://www.webmd.com/>.

"WHO | World Health Organization." WHO | World Health Organization. Web. 2014. <http://www.who.int/en/>.